# DIMENSIONAL APPROACHES IN DIAGNOSTIC CLASSIFICATION

*Refining the Research Agenda
for DSM-V*

# DIMENSIONAL APPROACHES IN DIAGNOSTIC CLASSIFICATION

*Refining the Research Agenda
for DSM-V*

Edited by

**John E. Helzer, M.D.**
**Helena Chmura Kraemer, Ph.D.**
**Robert F. Krueger, Ph.D.**
**Hans-Ulrich Wittchen, Ph.D.**
**Paul J. Sirovatka, M.S.**
**Darrel A. Regier, M.D., M.P.H.**

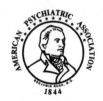

Published by the
American Psychiatric Association
Arlington, Virginia

**Note:** The authors have worked to ensure that all information in this book is accurate at the time of publication and consistent with general psychiatric and medical standards, and that information concerning drug dosages, schedules, and routes of administration is accurate at the time of publication and consistent with standards set by the U.S. Food and Drug Administration and the general medical community. As medical research and practice continue to advance, however, therapeutic standards may change. Moreover, specific situations may require a specific therapeutic response not included in this book. For these reasons and because human and mechanical errors sometimes occur, we recommend that readers follow the advice of physicians directly involved in their care or the care of a member of their family.

The findings, opinions, and conclusions of this report do not necessarily represent the views of the officers, trustees, or all members of the American Psychiatric Association. The views expressed are those of the authors of the individual chapters.

Copyright © 2008 American Psychiatric Association
ALL RIGHTS RESERVED

Manufactured in the United States of America on acid-free paper
12  11  10  09  08      5  4  3  2  1
First Edition

Typeset in Adobe's Frutiger and AGaramond.

American Psychiatric Association
1000 Wilson Boulevard
Arlington, VA 22209-3901
www.psych.org

**Library of Congress Cataloging-in-Publication Data**
Dimensional approaches in diagnostic classification : refining the research agenda for DSM-V / edited by John Helzer ... [et al.].
     p. ; cm.
   Includes bibliographical references and index.
   ISBN 978-0-89042-343-1 (alk. paper)
   1. Diagnostic and statistical manual of mental disorders. 2. Mental illness—Classification. 3. Mental illness—Diagnosis. I. Helzer, John E. II. American Psychiatric Association. [DNLM: 1. Diagnostic and statistical manual of mental disorders. 5th ed. 2. Mental Disorders—diagnosis. 3. Mental Disorders—classification. 4. Research. WM 141 D582 2008]
  RC455.2.C4D56 2008
  616.89'075—dc22

                                                          2008011900

**British Library Cataloguing in Publication Data**
A CIP record is available from the British Library.

This monograph is dedicated to Paul J. Sirovatka, whose untimely death in September 2007 deprived the American Psychiatric Association and the larger mental health community of an outstanding science writer and colleague. His long career at the National Institute of Mental Health and his many contributions to the development of the DSM-V revision are honored by our dedication of this volume of our research development series to Paul.

# CONTENTS

# CONTRIBUTORS

Thomas M. Achenbach, Ph.D.
Professor of Psychiatry and Psychology, Department of Psychiatry, University of Vermont, Burlington, Vermont

Judith Allardyce, M.B., Ch.B., MRCPsych, CCST
Researcher, Department of Psychiatry and Neuropsychology, South Limburg Mental Health Research and Teaching Network, EURON, Maastricht University, Maastricht, The Netherlands

Robert R. Althoff, M.D.
Assistant Professor of Psychiatry and Pediatrics, Department of Psychiatry, University of Vermont, Burlington, Vermont

Gavin Andrews, M.D.
Director and Scientia Professor of Psychiatry, Clinical Research Unit for Anxiety and Depression, University of New South Wales at St. Vincent's Hospital, Sydney, Australia

Katja Beesdo, Ph.D.
Research Fellow, Institute of Clinical Psychology and Psychotherapy, Technische Universität Dresden, Dresden, Germany

Ingvar Bjelland, M.D., Ph.D.
Specialist in Psychiatry and Child and Adolescent Psychiatry, Clinic for Child and Adolescent Mental Health Services, Haukeland University Hospital, Bergen, Norway

James P. Breiling, Ph.D.
Program Chief, Psychopathology, Behavioral Dysregulation, and Measurement Development Research Program, Division of Adult Translational Research and Treatment Development, National Institute of Mental Health, Bethesda, Maryland

Traolach Brugha, M.D.
Professor of Psychiatry and Director of Research, Department of Health Sciences, Clinical Division of Psychiatry, University of Leicester, Leicester, United Kingdom

**Kathleen K. Bucholz, Ph.D.**
Professor of Psychiatry, Department of Psychiatry and Midwest Alcoholism Research Center, Washington University School of Medicine, St. Louis, Missouri

**Wilson M. Compton, M.D., M.P.E.**
Director, Division of Epidemiology, Services, and Prevention Research, National Institute on Drug Abuse, Bethesda, Maryland

**Farifteh Firoozmand Duffy, Ph.D.**
Research Scientist, American Psychiatric Institute for Research and Education, Arlington, Virginia

**Andrew T. Gloster, Ph.D.**
Assistant Professor of Clinical Psychology and Psychotherapy, Institute of Clinical Psychology and Psychotherapy, Technische Universität Dresden, Dresden, Germany

**Michael Gossop, Ph.D.**
Professor, National Addiction Centre, Institute of Psychiatry, King's College London, and Head of Research, Addiction, Maudsley Hospital, London, United Kingdom

**Bridget F. Grant, Ph.D.**
Chief, Laboratory of Epidemiology and Biometry, Division of Clinical and Biological Research, National Institute on Alcohol Abuse and Alcoholism, Rockville, Maryland

**John E. Helzer, M.D.**
Professor of Psychiatry and Director, Health Behavior Research Center, University of Vermont College of Medicine, Burlington, Vermont

**Yueqin Huang, M.D., M.P.H., Ph.D.**
Professor of Psychiatric Epidemiology and Deputy Director, Institute of Mental Health, Peking University, Beijing, People's Republic of China

**James J. Hudziak, M.D.**
Professor, Psychiatry, Medicine, and Pediatrics and Director, Vermont Center for Children, Youth, and Families, University of Vermont College of Medicine, Burlington, Vermont; Thomas M. Achenbach Chair in Developmental Psychopathology, and Professor, Biological Psychology, Vrije University, Amsterdam, The Netherlands

**Helena Chmura Kraemer, Ph.D.**
Professor Emerita of Biostatistics in Psychiatry, Department of Psychiatry and Behavioral Sciences, Stanford University, Palo Alto, California

**Robert F. Krueger, Ph.D.**
Professor of Clinical Psychology, and Personality, Individual Differences, and Behavior Genetics, Department of Psychology, University of Minnesota, Minneapolis, Minnesota

**W. John Livesley, M.D., Ph.D.**
Professor Emeritus, Department of Psychiatry, Faculty of Medicine, University of British Columbia, Vancouver, British Columbia, Canada

**Marsha F. Lopez, Ph.D., M.H.S.**
Health Scientist Administrator, Division of Epidemiology, Services, and Prevention Research, National Institute on Drug Abuse, Bethesda, Maryland

**Daniel S. Pine, M.D.**
Chief, Section on Development and Affective Neuroscience; Chief of Child and Adolescent Research, Mood and Anxiety Disorders Program, National Institute of Mental Health, Bethesda, Maryland

**Darrel A. Regier, M.D., M.P.H.**
Executive Director, American Psychiatric Institute for Research and Education; Director, Division of Research, American Psychiatric Association, Arlington, Virginia

**Paola Rucci, Ph.D.**
Research Assistant Professor of Psychiatry, University of Pittsburgh School of Medicine, Pittsburgh, Pennsylvania

**M. Katherine Shear, M.D.**
Marion E. Kenworthy Professor of Psychiatry in the Faculty of Social Work, Columbia University School of Social Work and Department of Psychiatry, Columbia University College of Physicians and Surgeons, New York, New York

**Patrick E. Shrout, Ph.D.**
Professor of Psychology, Department of Psychology, New York University, New York, New York

**Paul J. Sirovatka, M.S.**
Director, Research Policy Analysis, Division of Research and American Psychiatric Institute for Research and Education, American Psychiatric Association, Arlington, Virginia

Andrew E. Skodol, M.D.
President, Institute for Mental Health Research, Phoenix, Arizona; Research Professor, University of Arizona College of Medicine, Tucson, Arizona

Timothy Slade, Ph.D.
Research Fellow, Department of Psychiatry, Clinical Research Unit for Anxiety and Depression, University of New South Wales at St. Vincent's Hospital, Sydney, Australia

Trisha Suppes, M.D., Ph.D.
Professor of Psychiatry, Department of Psychiatry and Director, Bipolar Disorder Research Program, University of Texas Southwestern Medical Center, Dallas, Texas

Michael E. Thase, M.D.
Professor of Psychiatry, University of Pennsylvania School of Medicine and Philadelphia Veterans Affairs Medical Center, Philadelphia, Pennsylvania, and University of Pittsburgh Medical Center, Pittsburgh, Pennsylvania

Jim van Os, M.D.
Professor of Psychiatry, Department of Psychiatry and Neuropsychology, South Limburg Mental Health Research and Teaching Network, EURON, Maastricht University, Maastricht, The Netherlands; Visiting Professor, Division of Psychological Medicine, Institute of Psychiatry, London, United Kingdom

Hans-Ulrich Wittchen, Ph.D.
Director, Institute of Clinical Psychology and Psychotherapy, Technische Universität Dresden, Dresden, Germany

# DISCLOSURE STATEMENT

The research conference series that produced this monograph is supported with funding from the U.S. National Institutes of Health (NIH) Grant No. U13 - MH067855 (Principal Investigator: Darrel A. Regier, M.D., M.P.H.). The National Institute of Mental Health (NIMH), the National Institute on Drug Abuse (NIDA), and the National Institute on Alcohol Abuse and Alcoholism (NIAAA) jointly support this cooperative research planning conference project. The Workgroup/Conference on Dimensional Approaches in Diagnostic Classification is not part of the official revision process for the *Diagnostic and Statistical Manual of Mental Disorders,* Fifth Edition (DSM-V), but rather is a separate, rigorous research planning initiative meant to inform revisions of psychiatric diagnostic classification systems. No private-industry sources provide funding for this research review.

Coordination and oversight of the overall research review, publicly titled "The Future of Psychiatric Diagnosis: Refining the Research Agenda," are provided by an Executive Steering Committee composed of representatives of the several entities that are cooperatively sponsoring the NIH-funded project. Present and former members are as follows:

- *American Psychiatric Institute for Research and Education*—Darrel A. Regier, M.D., M.P.H.; support staff: William E. Narrow, M.D., M.P.H., Maritza Rubio-Stipec, Sci.D., Paul J. Sirovatka, M.S., Jennifer Shupinka, Rocio Salvador, and Kristin Edwards
- *World Health Organization*—Benedetto Saraceno, M.D., and Norman Sartorius, M.D., Ph.D. (consultant)
- *National Institutes of Health*—Michael Kozak, Ph.D. (NIMH), Wilson M. Compton, M.D. (NIDA), and Bridget F. Grant, Ph.D. (NIAAA); NIMH grant project officers have included Bruce Cuthbert, Ph.D., Lisa Colpe, Ph.D., Michael Kozak, Ph.D., and Karen H. Bourdon, M.A.
- *Columbia University*—Michael B. First, M.D. (consultant)

The following contributors to this book have indicated financial interests in or other affiliations with a commercial supporter, a manufacturer of a commercial product, a provider of a commercial service, a nongovernmental organization, and/or a government agency, as listed below:

*Darrel A. Regier, M.D., M.P.H.*—The author, as Executive Director of the American Psychiatric Institute for Research and Education (APIRE), oversees all federal and industry-sponsored research and research training grants in APIRE but receives no external salary funding or honoraria from any government or industry sources.

*M. Katherine Shear, M.D.*—The author has served as a consultant to Pfizer and Forest.

*Patrick E. Shrout, Ph.D.*—The author has consulted with Dr. Hector Bird at Columbia University, who intends to pay a small fee from a grant from McNeill Pediatrics, a Division of McNeill PPC, Inc. No oversight of work was provided or required.

*Andrew E. Skodol, M.D.*—The author has received grant support from NIMH.

*Trisha Suppes, M.D., Ph.D.*—The author is the process of resigning from all advisory boards and has served as a consultant for Abbott Laboratories, AstraZeneca, Eli Lilly Research Laboratories, GlaxoSmithKline Pharmaceuticals, Novartis Pharmaceuticals, and Pfizer Inc. She has served on the Speakers' Bureau for AstraZeneca and GlaxoSmithKline Pharmaceuticals. The author has received funding or medications for clinical grants from Abbott Laboratories, AstraZeneca, GlaxoSmithKline Pharmaceuticals, JDS Pharmaceuticals, Janssen Pharmaceutica, NIMH, Novartis Pharmaceuticals, Pfizer Inc., the Stanley Medical Research Institute, and Wyeth. She receives royalties from Compact Clinicals.

*Michael E. Thase, M.D.*—The author has served as a consultant to AstraZeneca, Bristol-Myers Squibb Company, Cephalon, Inc., Cyberonics, Inc., Eli Lilly & Co., GlaxoSmithKline, Janssen Pharmaceutica, MedAvante, Inc., Neuronetics, Inc., Novartis, Organon, Inc., Sepracor, Inc., Shire US Inc., and Wyeth Pharmaceuticals. He has served on the Speakers' Bureau for AstraZeneca, Bristol-Myers Squibb Company, Cyberonics, Inc., Eli Lilly & Co., GlaxoSmithKline, Organon, Inc., Sanofi Aventis, and Wyeth Pharmaceuticals. He has equity holdings in MedAvante, Inc. The author receives royalties from American Psychiatric Publishing, Inc., Guilford Publications, and Herald House.

The following contributors to this book do not have any conflicts of interest to disclose:

Thomas M. Achenbach, Ph.D.
Judith Allardyce, M.B., Ch.B., MRCPsych, CCST
Robert R. Althoff, M.D.
Gavin Andrews, M.D.
Katja Beesdo, Ph.D.
Ingvar Bjelland, M.D., Ph.D.
James P. Breiling, Ph.D.
Traolach Brugha, M.D.
Kathleen K. Bucholz, Ph.D.
Wilson M. Compton, M.D., M.P.E.
Farifteh Firoozmand Duffy, Ph.D.
Andrew T. Gloster, Ph.D.
Michael Gossop, Ph.D.
Bridget F. Grant, Ph.D.
John E. Helzer, M.D.
Yueqin Huang, M.D., M.P.H., Ph.D.
James J. Hudziak, M.D.
Helena Chmura Kraemer, Ph.D.
Robert F. Krueger, Ph.D.
W. John Livesley, M.D., Ph.D.
Marsha F. Lopez, Ph.D., M.H.S.
Daniel S. Pine, M.D.
Paola Rucci, Ph.D.
Timothy Slade, Ph.D.
Jim van Os, M.D.
Hans-Ulrich Wittchen, Ph.D.

# FOREWORD

## Dimensional Approaches to Psychiatric Classification

Darrel A. Regier, M.D., M.P.H.

We are pleased to have the opportunity to present in this book a selection of contributions, first published as articles in a supplement to the *International Journal of Methods in Psychiatric Research,* that report the proceedings of a conference focused on dimensional approaches to psychiatric diagnosis. Convened by the American Psychiatric Association (APA) in collaboration with the World Health Organization (WHO) and the U.S. National Institutes of Health (NIH), with funding provided by the NIH, the conference was one in a series titled "The Future of Psychiatric Diagnosis: Refining the Research Agenda."

## Research Planning for DSM/ICD

The APA/WHO/NIH conference series represents a key element in a multiphase research review process designed to set the stage for the fifth revision of the *Diagnostic and Statistical Manual of Mental Disorders* (DSM-V). In its entirety, the project entails 10 workgroups, each focused on a specific diagnostic topic or category, and two additional workgroups dedicated to methodological considerations in nosology and classification. APA attaches high priority to ensuring that information and research recommendations generated by each of the workgroups are readily available to scientific groups who are concurrently updating other national and international classifications of mental and behavioral disorders.

---

Reprinted with permission from Regier DA. "Dimensional Approaches to Psychiatric Classification: Refining the Research Agenda for DSM-V: An Introduction." *International Journal of Methods in Psychiatric Research* 2007; 16(S1): S1–S5.

Within the APA, the American Psychiatric Institute for Research and Education (APIRE), under the direction of Darrel A. Regier, M.D., M.P.H., holds lead responsibility for organizing and administering the diagnosis research planning conferences. Members of the Executive Steering Committee for the series include representatives of the WHO's Division of Mental Health and Prevention of Substance Abuse and of three NIH components that are jointly funding the project: the National Institute of Mental Health (NIMH), the National Institute on Drug Abuse (NIDA), and the National Institute on Alcohol Abuse and Alcoholism (NIAAA).

The APA published the fourth edition of DSM in 1994 (American Psychiatric Association 1994) and a text revision in 2000 (American Psychiatric Association 2000). Although DSM-V is not scheduled to appear until 2012, planning for the fifth revision began in 1999 with collaboration between the APA and NIMH designed to stimulate research that would address identified opportunities in psychiatric nosology. A first product of this joint venture was preparation of six white papers that proposed broad-brush recommendations for research in key areas; topics included developmental issues, gaps in the current classification, disability and impairment, neuroscience, nomenclature, and cross-cultural issues. Each team that developed a paper included at least one liaison member from NIMH, with the intent—largely realized—that these members would integrate many of the workgroups' recommendations into NIMH research support programs. These white papers were published in *A Research Agenda for DSM-V* (Kupfer et al. 2002). This volume more recently has been followed by a second compilation of white papers (Narrow et al. 2007) that outline diagnosis-related research needs in the areas of gender, infants and children, and geriatric populations.

As a second phase of planning, the APA leadership envisioned a series of international research planning conferences that would address specific diagnostic topics in greater depth, with conference proceedings serving as resource documents for groups involved in the official DSM-V revision process. A prototype symposium on mood disorders was held in conjunction with the XII World Congress of Psychiatry in Yokohama, Japan, in late 2002. Presentations addressed diverse topics in depression-related research, including established reliability and clinical utility of prior DSM preclinical animal models, genetics, pathophysiology, functional imaging, clinical treatment, epidemiology, prevention, medical comorbidity, and public health implications of the classification issues across the full spectrum of mood disorders. This pilot meeting underscored the importance of structuring multi-disciplinary research planning conferences in a manner that would force interaction among investigators from different fields and elicit a sharp focus on the diagnostic implications of recent and planned research. Lessons learned in Yokohama guided development of a proposal for the cooperative research planning conference grant that NIMH awarded to APIRE in 2003, with substantial additional funding support from NIDA and NIAAA. The conferences funded under the grant are the basis for this monograph series and represent a second major phase in the scientific review and planning for DSM-V.

Finally, a third component of advance planning has been the DSM-V Prelude Project, an APA-sponsored web site designed to keep the DSM user community and the public informed about research and other activities related to the fifth revision of the manual. An "outreach" section of the site permits interested parties to submit comments about problems with DSM-IV and suggestions for DSM-V. All submissions are being entered into the DSM-V Prelude database for eventual referral to the appropriate DSM-V workgroups. This site and associated links can be accessed at www.dsm5.org.

The conferences that comprise the core activity of the second phase of preparation have multiple objectives. One is to promote international collaboration among members of the scientific community with the aim of eliminating the remaining disparities between DSM-V and the International Classification of Diseases (World Health Organization 1992b) Mental and Behavioural Disorders section (World Health Organization 1992a). The WHO has launched the revision of ICD-10 that will lead to publication of the 11th edition in approximately 2014. A second goal is to stimulate the empirical research necessary to allow informed decision-making regarding deficiencies identified in DSM-IV. A third is to facilitate the development of broadly agreed upon criteria that researchers worldwide can use in planning and conducting future research exploring the etiology and pathophysiology of mental disorders. Challenging as it is, this last objective reflects widespread agreement in the field that the well-established reliability and clinical utility of prior DSM classifications must be matched in the future by a renewed focus on the validity of diagnoses.

Given the vision of an ultimately unified international system for classifying mental disorders, members of the Executive Steering Committee have attached high priority to assuring the participation of investigators from all parts of the world in the project. Toward this end, each conference in the series has two co-chairs, drawn respectively from the United States (U.S.) and a country other than the U.S.; approximately half of the experts invited to each working conference are from outside the U.S.; and half of the conferences are being convened outside the U.S.

# Toward Dimensional Approaches: A Historical Perspective

Establishing a workgroup, and convening a conference, on dimensional approaches to psychiatric diagnosis reflects both a long-term interest of nosologists throughout the world and an immediate outcome the APA/WHO/NIH conference series. Under the co-chairmanship of Thomas A. Widiger and Erik Simonsen, the first workgroup in this project to convene a conference focused on dimensional approaches to personality disorders, conditions long considered prime candidates for a dimensional or quantitative approach to assessment and diagnosis. Papers presented at the meeting were published in two successive issues of the *Journal of Personality Disorders* (Vol. 19, Nos. 2 and 3, 2005; a full collection of papers presented at the meeting was published in the initial monograph in this series) (Widiger et al. 2006).

While personality disorders underscore the potential value of incorporating dimensional approaches into the existing categorical, or binary, classification of DSM, diagnoses that have been the focus of other workgroups have made evident broad interest within the profession in the feasibility and potential benefits of incorporating a dimensional component to the diagnosis of all psychiatric, including addictive, disorders.

Absent an understanding of the causal mechanisms of mental disorders or of the specifics of brain or behavioral mechanisms gone awry, throughout much of the last century, psychiatry—American psychiatry, certainly—grounded claims for the validity of psychiatric disorder diagnoses on the presumed etiology of mental disorders as reactions either to unconscious conflicts or to known or putative environmental stressors, for the most part in the absence of empirical research. The publication by Robins and Guze (1970) of a radically new proposal for a research-based approach to validity marked a decisive turning point in the U.S. approach to psychiatric nosology as embodied theretofore in the American Psychiatric Association's *Diagnostic and Statistical Manual of Mental Disorders* (DSM), first (American Psychiatric Association 1952) and second (American Psychiatric Association 1968) editions. That seminal paper spurred growing interest in developing a nosology that would take an atheoretical position with respect to etiology and, rather than assert validity, would emphasize first the reliability of diagnoses through a focus on identifying syndromes and defining explicit criteria capable of being observed and replicated across settings. The Feighner criteria (Feighner et al. 1972) represented an initial response to the challenge of Robins and Guze to develop highly specific phenomenological descriptions of disorders, with a tacit expectation that such descriptions would result in phenomenological subtypes that would eventually correlate with etiological and pathophysiological factors needed to validate these more precise clinical syndromes.

The pieces of this optimistic vision failed to fall neatly into place when nosologists were confronted with the reality of patient populations who, while appearing to have similar clinical presentations, proved to be highly heterogeneous. The strategy chosen to deal with this sobering reality entailed the introduction, in DSM-III (American Psychiatric Association 1980), of a polythetic—or, more descriptively, a Chinese menu—approach wherein the existence of a disorder would be based on the presence of a certain number—e.g., at least five of nine possible—of criteria that reliably sorted a wide range of individuals into broad diagnostic categories. Nonetheless, because of the feasibility of multiple combinations of criteria, some heterogeneity is inevitably introduced into these broad categories.

While the criteria in DSM-III were intended as hypotheses that necessarily were subject to empirical testing, they also were quickly incorporated into key diagnostic assessment instruments, such as the Diagnostic Interview Schedule (DIS; Robins et al. 1981), and taken into the field in the landmark Epidemiologic Catchment Area (ECA; Regier et al. 1984) study. The ECA found unexpectedly high comorbidity between so-called primary disorders higher on a diagnostic hierarchy such as schizophrenia and other disorders listed in the exclusion criteria, such as panic disorder. The failure of DSM-III criteria to specifically define individuals with only one disorder served as an alert that the strict neo-Kraepelinian categorical approach to mental disorder diagnoses advocated by Robins and Guze (1970), Spitzer et al. (1978), and others could have some serious problems. Many years later, in a trenchant critique of implicit "disease entity" validity criteria championed in the 1970s, Kendall and Jablensky (2003) pointed out that Robins and Guze, and others, simply had failed to consider the possibility that "…disorders might merge into one another with no natural boundary in between." Indeed, early recognition of this problem had led to dropping diagnostic hierarchies from the revised third edition of DSM (DSM-III-R; American Psychiatric Association 1987).

Lessons learned which led to DSM-III-R—i.e., that a polythetic approach to determining the presence or absence of a disorder would inevitably identify as positive for illness individuals with little impairment or distress—had far-reaching reverberations that eventuated, in DSM-IV, in the introduction of a clinical significance criterion within mental disorder criteria sets. Far from being unanimously agreed to, this innovation prompted objections on the part of many who viewed the clinical significance criterion as imprecise. The dissatisfaction led to calls for a greater number of required criteria, as prerequisites for diagnosis, and, alternatively, for collection of contextual information that would aid in diagnosis. Such informational needs, as we see in the chapters presented in this volume, now are increasingly perceived to require the incorporation of a dimensional component to the classification system.

In the 27 years since introduction of DSM-III, the research enterprise has been instrumental in advancing the use of dimensional measures. While debate continues among nosologists regarding use of dimensional criteria to ascertain the threshold or severity of mental disorders in the clinical setting, physician scientists are routinely reliant on rating instruments that are inherently dimensional to assess severity or treatment response in clinical trials.

As the APA begins the process of research, evaluation, and analysis that will eventuate in publication of DSM-V in 2012, the chapters presented in this book document perspectives on the issue in 2007. We hope that the ideas presented here stimulate interest in finding new ways of combining categorical and dimensional approaches.

# Acknowledgments

Four leaders in the field—John E. Helzer, M.D., University of Vermont; Helena Kraemer, Ph.D., Stanford University; Robert Krueger, Ph.D., University of Minnesota; and Hans-Ulrich Wittchen, M.D., Technische Universität Dresden—agreed to organize and co-chair the "Dimensional Approaches to Psychiatric Classification" workgroup and conference, which convened in Bethesda, Maryland, in July 2006. The co-chairs worked closely with the APA/WHO/NIH Executive Steering Committee to identify and enlist a stellar roster of participants for the conference.

We appreciate the enthusiastic interest of Dr. Wittchen, editor-in-chief of the *International Journal of Methods in Psychiatric Research,* in ensuring the availability of these papers to a global readership. In addition, a summary report of the conference is available on-line at www.dsm5.org.

We express our appreciation to officials at NIMH, NIDA, and NIAAA who made supplementary funding available to convene the workgroup on dimensional approaches and thus to stimulate future research on this vital topic. The APA greatly appreciates, as well, the contributions of all participants in the dimensional approaches research planning workgroup and the interest of our broader audience in this topic.

# References

American Psychiatric Association. Diagnostic and Statistical Manual: Mental Disorders. Washington, DC: American Psychiatric Association, 1952.

American Psychiatric Association. Diagnostic and Statistical Manual of Mental Disorders, 2nd Edition. Washington, DC: American Psychiatric Association, 1968.

American Psychiatric Association. Diagnostic and Statistical Manual of Mental Disorders, 3rd Edition. Washington, DC: American Psychiatric Association, 1980.

American Psychiatric Association. Diagnostic and Statistical Manual of Mental Disorders, 3rd Edition, Revised. Washington, DC: American Psychiatric Association, 1987.

American Psychiatric Association. Diagnostic and Statistical Manual of Mental Disorders, 4th Edition. Washington, DC: American Psychiatric Association, 1994.

American Psychiatric Association. Diagnostic and Statistical Manual of Mental Disorders, 4th Edition, Text Revision. Washington, DC: American Psychiatric Association, 2000.

Feighner JF, Robins E, Guze SB, et al. Diagnostic criteria for use in psychiatric research. Arch Gen Psychiatry 1972; 26: 57–63.

Kendall R, Jablensky A. Distinguishing between the validity and utility of psychiatric diagnoses. Am J Psychiatry 2003; 160: 2–12.

Kupfer DJ, First MB, Regier DA (eds). A Research Agenda for DSM-V. Washington, DC: American Psychiatric Association, 2002.

Narrow WE, First MB, Sirovatka P, Regier DA (eds). Age and Gender Considerations in Psychiatric Diagnosis: A Research Agenda for DSM-V. Arlington, VA: American Psychiatric Association, 2007.

Regier DA, Meyer JK, Kramer M, et al. The NIMH Epidemiologic Catchment Area program: historical context, major objectives, and study population characteristics. Arch Gen Psychiatry 1984; 41: 934–941.

Robins E, Guze SB. Establishment of diagnostic validity in psychiatric illness: its application to schizophrenia. Am J Psychiatry 1970; 126: 983–987.

Robins LN, Helzer JE, Croughan J, et al. National Institute of Mental Health Diagnostic Interview Schedule: its history, characteristics, and validity. Arch Gen Psychiatry 1981; 38: 381–389.

Spitzer RL, Endicott J, Robins E. Research Diagnostic Criteria: rationale and reliability. Arch Gen Psychiatry 1978; 35: 773–782.

Widiger TA, Simonsen E, Sirovatka PJ, Regier DA. Dimensional Models of Personality Disorders: Refining the Research Agenda for DSM-V. Washington, DC: American Psychiatric Association, 2006.

World Health Organization. The ICD-10 Classification of Mental and Behavioural Disorders: Clinical Descriptions and Diagnostic Guidelines. Geneva: World Health Organization, 1992a.

World Health Organization. International Statistical Classification of Diseases and Related Health Problems, 10th Revision. Geneva: World Health Organization, 1992b.

# PREFACE

John E. Helzer, M.D.

If you do not know the name of things, the knowledge of them is lost too.

Carl Linnaeus (1707–1778)

The third edition of the *Diagnostic and Statistical Manual of Mental Disorders* (DSM-III; American Psychiatric Association) revolutionized psychiatric diagnosis when it was published in 1980. DSM-III and its subsequent revisions have fostered dramatic progress in psychiatric taxonomy. The manuals have provided a process for harnessing the collective wisdom of the field to create illness definitions; a consistent diagnostic language for clinical work, research, and teaching; improved patient and public communication about mental illness; and a common international taxonomic standard (Kendell and Jablensky 2003). Structured and semi-structured assessment tools based on these definitions are now the research standard for mental disorders. Explicit diagnostic criteria like those contained in DSM enable us to achieve diagnostic reliability comparable to X rays and EKGs (Helzer et al. 1977). And by improving reliability, they have raised the lower bound for validity.

But, as articulated by Kupfer et al. in their volume *A Research Agenda for DSM-V* (2002), as useful as the DSM-III paradigm was, a new paradigm may be needed if we are to be successful in uncovering illness etiology in psychiatry. An important goal for the DSM-V research agenda is "to transcend the limitations of the current DSM paradigm and encourage a research agenda that goes beyond our current ways of thinking (about diagnosis)." (Kupfer et al. 2002, p. xix). The conference reported in this volume did exactly that. The challenge to the participants was to go beyond the current categorical illness definitions as set forth in DSM-III and DSM-IV and suggest ways of incorporating more quantitative, dimensional concepts into DSM-V.

As detailed in the chapters of this volume, categorical definitions of illness have inherent limitations. These limitations have long been recognized by the Task Forces and workgroups that have created and revised past editions of DSM. The introductions to each of the revisions have noted the provisional nature of the diagnostic definitions and the desirability of a more quantitative, dimensional approach. The potential advantages of quantitative assessment of mental illness have been well articulated and are reviewed by Helena Chmura Kraemer, one of the conference co-chairs, in this volume. Her endorsement of the need for both categorical and dimensional approaches is illustrated by the popularity, in both clinical and research contexts, of rating scales for quantifying illnesses once they have been diagnosed categorically. However, the struggle for the DSM committees has been, and will be, to find ways to create dimensional measures that are compatible with categorical definitions and not overly disruptive to clinical practice. The conference reported in this monograph was specifically intended to grapple with those issues.

## Organization of This Volume

In his Foreword, Darrel Regier reviews the research planning process for DSM-V and details the background of this conference on dimensional approaches to diagnosis. In Chapter 1, by Lopez et al., representatives from each of the NIH institutes that joined with APIRE in providing scientific and financial support for the conference express the hope that this volume will address the following issues: 1) how to create and apply dimensional measures to specific disorders, 2) how dimensional approaches can enhance diagnostic precision, 3) the co-occurrence of psychiatric disorders, 4) syndrome thresholds, and 5) the feasibility of applying dimensional measures in clinical settings. These issues and others are all discussed in this volume.

In Chapter 2, "DSM Categories and Dimensions in Clinical and Research Contexts," Kraemer discusses the intellectual foundation for a dimensional classification, details the relative advantages and potential drawbacks of both categorical and dimensional approaches, and argues that both should be utilized in DSM-V. The six subsequent chapters are organized by diagnostic area, including substance use, affective, psychotic, anxiety, personality, and developmental disorders. Each chapter provides examples of the constraints of a purely categorical approach to diagnosis and offers ideas for integrating a dimensional equivalent that can be related back to the categorical definitions. In the final chapter, the conference co-chairs summarize key points in each of the other chapters and highlight particular topics, such as cross-cutting dimensions, sensitivity to developmental issues, and relevance of dimensional approaches for clinicians. They conclude with a simple proposal for a dimensional option in DSM-V that would address problems raised in the other chapters, and final thoughts on structuring DSM-V to anticipate future diagnostic needs.

# References

American Psychiatric Association. Diagnostic and Statistical Manual of Mental Disorders, 3rd Edition. Washington, DC: American Psychiatric Association, 1980.

Helzer JE, Clayton PJ, Pambakian R, Reich T, Woodruff RA Jr, Reveley MA. Reliability of psychiatric diagnosis. II. The test/retest reliability of diagnostic classification. Arch Gen Psychiatry 1977; 34: 136–41.

Kendell R, Jablensky A. Distinguishing between the validity and utility of psychiatric diagnoses. Am J Psychiatry 2003; 160: 4–12.

Kupfer DJ, First MB, Regier DA (eds). A Research Agenda for DSM-V. Washington, DC: American Psychiatric Association, 2002.

# 1

# DIMENSIONAL APPROACHES IN DIAGNOSTIC CLASSIFICATION

## A Critical Appraisal

Marsha F. Lopez, Ph.D., M.H.S.
Wilson M. Compton, M.D., M.P.E.
Bridget F. Grant, Ph.D.
James P. Breiling, Ph.D.

Clinicians and researchers alike struggle to diagnose psychiatric conditions in a manner that is etiologically and therapeutically meaningful. The *Diagnostic and Statistical Manual of Mental Disorders* (DSM) system as it currently exists falls short of achieving these goals because without satisfactory grounding in etiology, any diagnostic rubric will remain suboptimal. In the meantime, after decades of categorical approaches to psychiatric disorder through DSM, science is considering a shift toward integrating new dimensional applications with the current categorical approaches.

The papers reprinted in this book represent a collaboration among the National Institute on Drug Abuse, the National Institute on Alcohol Abuse and Al-

Reprinted with permission from Lopez MF, Compton WM, Grant BF, Breiling JP. "Dimensional Approaches in Diagnostic Classification: A Critical Appraisal." *International Journal of Methods in Psychiatric Research* 2007; 16(S1): S6–S7.

coholism, the National Institute of Mental Health, and the American Psychiatric Association to address questions and issues related to dimensional aspects of specific diagnostic areas, including a review of the existing research and clinical practices and development of an agenda for future investigation. Regardless of whether the recommendations of these workgroups will result in the introduction of dimensional approaches into DSM-V, the ultimate goal is to improve clinical research and apply gained knowledge to reduce disability and burden from psychiatric illness.

Psychiatry is at a crossroads with DSM-V. Research and clinical practitioners seek to determine whether the field is ready for diagnoses based on continuous measures of psychopathology. This readiness exists on at least two levels. First, there is clear evidence that psychiatric disorders can be measured dimensionally. Second, this evidence offers promise for translation into clinical decision-making. With recent innovations in statistical methods and research practices, it has become clear that psychopathology can be viewed not only as absent or present, but dimensionally, via measures such as frequency and severity that can assist in determining a therapeutic path (Kessler 2002; Krueger et al. 2005; Saha et al. 2006). Yet, despite convincing research findings, clinicians face a difficult problem in determining the point at which a patient is in need of treatment or follow-up care. The cut points stipulated in the current DSM system determine who does and who does not receive a diagnosis, and who does and does not receive treatment.

Complicating matters, readiness of the field for dimensional diagnostic approaches is not consistent across all the psychiatric disorders represented in DSM. For example, in the case of substance use disorders, measures of frequency of use provide a relatively straightforward way to incorporate a severity dimension, whereas psychoses do not have a convenient analogous proxy for severity. That example does not demonstrate that psychoses cannot be measured in a dimensional fashion, but it illustrates a difficulty to be addressed in considering a shift from exclusively categorical definitions of psychiatric disorders to more continuous measures of psychopathology.

Leaders in research and clinical practice of psychiatry gathered to confront questions of readiness for and feasibility of dimensional diagnoses, and these chapters are a product of those discussions. We hope that this volume addresses several important issues: (1) how to create and apply dimensional measures to specific disorders, (2) how dimensional approaches can enhance diagnostic precision, (3) the co-occurrence of psychiatric disorders, (4) syndrome thresholds, and (5) feasibility of applying dimensional measures in clinical settings. In addition, a major objective is to identify ways of incorporating developmental, demographic, and genetic findings into the threshold models. A goal is to determine the appropriateness of blending dimensional and categorical approaches and to provide disorder-specific recommendations for their integration.

We at the National Institutes of Health are excited to see these issues addressed after years of discussion in meetings and the literature. Although psychiatry may not be currently able to incorporate dimensional aspects of diagnosis throughout DSM-V, it is certainly ready to consider the implications of such major changes in the approach to classification. Our hope is that the resulting recommendations will transform psychiatric research and practice such that advancements in identifying, preventing, and treating psychopathology will improve mental health and addiction outcomes worldwide.

## References

Kessler RC. The categorical versus dimensional assessment controversy in the sociology of mental illness. J Health Soc Behav 2002; 43(2): 171–188.

Krueger RF, Watson D, Barlow DH. Introduction to the special section: toward a dimensionally based taxonomy of psychopathology. J Abnorm Psychol 2005; 114(4):491–493; and subsequent articles.

Saha TD, Chou SP, Grant BF. Toward an alcohol use disorder continuum using item response theory: results from the National Epidemiologic Survey on Alcohol and Related Conditions. Psychol Med 2006; 36(7): 931–941.

# 2

# DSM CATEGORIES AND DIMENSIONS IN CLINICAL AND RESEARCH CONTEXTS

Helena Chmura Kraemer, Ph.D.

The *Diagnostic and Statistical Manual of Mental Disorders* (DSM) has long provided standard diagnostic guidelines for both the clinical and research use in psychiatry, although not without substantial criticisms. Some of the criticisms are certainly warranted, since DSM continues to be a work in progress rather than a finished instrument. Some, however, arise because of semantic problems of which those seeking to develop DSM-V in the years to come must be aware.

DSM concerns "diagnoses," not "disorders." A "disorder" is something wrong in a patient that is of clinical relevance, a disease, a malfunction, an injury, an abnormality, etc., something problematic for the patient for which he or she would likely seek clinical attention and for which clinicians might provide effective treatment. DSM focus and concern has always been on "diagnoses," that is, a clinical expert's opinion as to whether some disorder is present in a particular patient. A diagnosis is to a disorder as is a sample to the population it represents, or a measure to the construct it is meant to assess; that is, a representation or an indication, not the goal itself. When users forget the possibility of sampling error inherent in a sample, or the measurement errors in a measure, results can mislead. In the same

Reprinted with permission from Kraemer HC. "DSM Categories and Dimensions in Clinical and Research Contexts." *International Journal of Methods in Psychiatric Research* 2007; 16(S1): S8–S15.

way, to date no diagnosis is perfectly reliable and valid for its disorder. Ignoring that fact can result in misleading conclusions.

The purpose of any diagnostic system, such as DSM, is not to say what is "normal" or "abnormal," nor what is or is not "acceptable" in any society (Caplan 1995); nor is it an effort to "medicalize" society's problems nor to channel clients to psychiatrists rather than to clinical psychologists, sociologists, or other mental health providers (Kirk and Kutchins 1992). DSM does not concern "insanity," a legal rather than a medical term, and assuredly does not concern who is "crazy" or "mad," terms that are layman pejorative terms not necessarily related to mental health disorders. Such terms continue to stigmatize those with mental health problems and are a major factor in the less than adequate care that those with mental health problems continue to receive. Yet many of the criticisms of DSM use exactly those terms, e.g., "They Say You're Crazy: How the World's Most Powerful Psychiatrists Decide Who's Normal" (Caplan 1995).

The word "diagnostic" in DSM is clearly descriptive of its purpose to provide the best guidance currently available to identify those with a disorder. More puzzling is the word "statistical" in DSM. DSM-I (American Psychiatric Association 1952) and DSM-II (American Psychiatric Association 1968) were proposed for purposes related primarily to counting cases: How many of those in institutions were in this general category rather than another? Is the number of those in a certain category increasing or decreasing over time? For such purposes, then and now, categorical diagnoses were necessary.

However, starting with DSM-III (American Psychiatric Association 1980), it has been recognized that DSM diagnoses serve many other types of clinical and clinical research purposes as well. In the clinic, they serve purposes related to prevention, early identification, management, and assessment of improvement for individual patients. In clinical research, the diagnoses play important roles in seeking to understand etiology and course and to identify effective and cost-effective treatments, i.e., to provide the evidence for evidence-based clinical decision-making.

DSM is not designed or intended to further basic science (the development of scientific theories, research on tissues or animal models), whether that basic science is medical, psychological, or sociological. It is not designed, for example, to further current medical, psychological, or sociological theories about cognition, personality, or functioning, although clearly all three are central to DSM diagnoses. If and when such theories lead to evidence that would advance understanding of the etiology, identification, treatment, course, or prognosis, then those results should and would influence DSM. Thus basic science should be expected ultimately to drive DSM, not the other way around.

With such issues in mind, clearly the word "statistical" in DSM now takes on greater meaning, for a goal of DSM is to facilitate drawing correct statistical inferences from what is observed. In the clinic, that would mean correct inferences about choice of treatment, monitoring treatment response, and maintaining health. In clinical research, that would mean guidance on issues related to measurement, design, analysis, and clinical interpretation of research results in epidemiological studies, in medical test evaluation, and in randomized clinical trials.

Obviously, while DSM relates to diagnosis and not to disorder, the goals of DSM can be approached only if there are close relationships between diagnoses and disorders. Such relationships are generally described by the reliability and validity of the diagnosis applied to a given disorder. Technically, the reliability of a diagnosis is the percentage of the person-to-person variability in a given population that relates to the variance of the "true" values of the diagnosis (Lord and Novick 1968). Less technically, it relates to the extent to which a second independent diagnostic opinion about a patient agrees with the first, and it is best measured by the correlation coefficient between independent test–retest diagnoses for a sample of subjects from that population.

Validity, however, is the percentage of the person-to-person variability of the diagnosis in a given population that relates to the variance of the disease for which the diagnosis is meant, and it is consequently always lower than the reliability of a diagnosis (Lord and Novick 1968). To date, DSMs have focused solely on face or clinical validity, the assertion that the diagnosis corresponds to clinicians' subjective views of a disorder. This is a weak but necessary form of validity achieved by requiring consensus among clinicians expert in that disorder, and such consensus has to date been the primary basis of DSM modifications. Ideally the validity of a diagnosis represents the correlation between the diagnosis and a "gold standard" determination of the disorder. For example, one common form of validity is expressed by the sensitivity and specificity of a categorical diagnosis relative to its corresponding disorder, where sensitivity is the probability that a person who has the disorder is diagnosed positive, and specificity is the probability that a person who does not have the disorder is diagnosed negative. However, in the absence of a "gold standard" diagnosis to serve as a criterion against which the diagnosis is tested, this is not yet possible for DSM, nor is it possible for most medical diagnoses.

In the absence of a "gold standard," establishing validity means challenging the validity using a variety of external criteria. The more such challenges a DSM diagnosis can withstand, the more likely it is to be valid. For example, if those with a certain diagnosis have a subsequent course similar to each other and quite different from those without that diagnosis, this is a type of predictive validity. If those with a certain diagnosis have a different genetic profile, are exposed to different environmental conditions, have a different characteristic brain structure and/or functioning, or respond differently to treatment than those without, each such demonstration provides increasing support for the validity of the diagnosis. If those with a diagnosis respond to certain interventions and not to others, that also is support for the validity of the diagnosis (Robins and Barrett 1989; Robins and Guze 1970).

Since DSM-III, major emphasis has been on test–retest reliability for three major reasons. First, reliability is easily assessed in practice, while, in the absence of a "gold standard" determining the presence or absence of the relevant disorder, establishing validity is a long and difficult process. Second, since the reliability of a diagnosis sets the ceiling for its validity, validity requires adequate reliability. Kirk and Kutchins (1992) criticized DSM because of this focus, suggesting that the development of the kappa as a measure of reliability had somehow derailed the diagnostic development process by focusing interest solely on reliability. This ignored the fact that another form of kappa serves as a primary measure of validity (Kraemer et al. 2002). Nevertheless, their criticism of the exclusive focus to date on reliability is valid and motivates increased efforts to challenge the validity of the diagnoses in future DSM development. Finally, it is well known that unreliability attenuates effect sizes and decreases the power of statistical tests, both of which compromise the ability of research to provide the evidence necessary to validate the diagnosis or to guide modifications to DSM (Kraemer and Thiemann 1987, 1989; Kraemer 1991).

The process of DSM development is analogous to a spiral (Kupfer and Thase 1989): A DSM version is proposed, which leads to clinical use and research applications that generate information on the reliability and validity of that diagnosis, which information is then used as a basis for the formulation of the next DSM version, and the process goes around again and again. Each successive iteration is expected to move closer to the true disorder. Where DSM-I and DSM-II focused on clinical validity, and DSM-III emphasized reliability, DSM-IV (American Psychiatric Association 1994) began to emphasize an evidence-based approach to diagnosis. DSM-V would be expected to do all this and more.

We propose one enhancement to DSM for DSM-V, one there is reason to believe would enhance both the reliability and validity of DSM diagnoses: the addition of a dimensional adjunct to each of the traditional categorical diagnoses of DSM. Including a corresponding dimensional scale along with a categorical diagnosis in DSM-V has nothing to do with the nature of disorders, and everything to do with the quality of a diagnosis for that disorder and for the clinical and research needs that such a diagnosis might serve. DSM's exclusive focus so far on categorical diagnosis is a historical fact stemming from the goals of the earliest DSMs. As the goals of DSM have broadened, the need for a corresponding dimensional approach has become more urgent.

In what follows we will first define the concepts on which this dimensional proposal is based. Then we will show a theoretical and a practical demonstration of the potential effects of this proposal, discuss possible objections, and consider right and wrong ways to implement the proposal.

## Categorical and Dimensional Diagnosis

A categorical diagnosis (at least in the way that term is used in DSM) has only two values: The patient is either positive (thought to have the disorder) or negative (thought not to have the disorder). Generally a categorical measure is one with two or more discrete non-ordered responses, and, technically, DSM uses binary diagnoses, but to avoid confusion we will continue to use the term most often used: categorical diagnosis.

A dimensional scale in contrast has three or more ordered values. Thus a three-point scale (e.g., 0, none; 1, some; or 2, severe symptoms) is dimensional (although little better than a categorical diagnosis), as is a 4, 5, 6, 7,… point scale (e.g., the Hamilton Depression Scale), a discrete score (e.g., number of drinks per week), or a continuum (e.g., body mass index, duration of symptoms). Multivariate diagnoses are included here as well (e.g., the combination of age of onset, total duration, and severity of symptoms). Again, "dimensional" is perhaps here a misnomer, for what is proposed would better be described as "ordinal" (univariate or multivariate), but we will continue to use the usual term "dimensional."

What is being proposed for DSM-V is not to substitute dimensional scales for categorical diagnoses, but to add a dimensional option to the usual categorical diagnoses for DSM-V. While it has often been opined that clinicians want categorical diagnoses and researchers want dimensional ones, that is not precisely true (Kraemer and O'Hara 2004). To assess whether a patient is responding to treatment, clinicians value the information provided by dimensional approaches. To decide whether a patient is eligible for a research study, researchers typically rely on a categorical diagnosis. Thus, if a dimensional option is added, those clinicians and clinical researchers who need or prefer to use the categorical diagnoses in certain contexts would continue to do so. Where corresponding dimensional scales enhance clinical or research decision-making, those dimensions would become available in DSM-V.

## WHEN IS A DIMENSIONAL DIAGNOSIS UNNEEDED OR IMPOSSIBLE?

The brief answer: virtually never. The only situation in which a dimensional adjunct would not add quality to the categorical diagnosis for a disorder is when there is no meaningful clinical variation among those who are diagnosed positive on the categorical diagnosis and no meaningful clinical variation among those who are diagnosed negative on the categorical diagnosis.

Consider this: In the past, cancer treatments were often compared using the success rates. If one survived 5 years past diagnosis, one was a success; otherwise, a failure. What this categorical definition did was to equate surviving 5 years plus 1 day to surviving 50 years postdiagnosis, and to equate surviving 5 days postdiagnosis to surviving 5 years minus 1 day. However, those surviving 5 years plus 1 day were considered completely different from those surviving 5 years minus 1 day, as different as those surviving 50 years were from those surviving 5 days. To both patient and clinician that makes little practical sense. In more recent years, survival methods have been used instead of this categorical response, thus substituting a dimensional measure (time) for a categorical measure.

That illustrates the problem with every categorical DSM diagnosis. Among those who have the diagnosis, there is variation in precursors: genotype, environmental exposures, age of onset, pre-morbid physiological, psychological, behavioral, and emotional characteristics; in concomitants: specific symptomatology, severity, duration of episodes and remissions, response to treatments; and in consequences: disability, impairment, diminished quality of life, shortened life span. Those with the diagnosis differ from each other in many respects, but which of the many ways in which those with the disorder differ are clinically significant is the question important to DSM-V. Similarly, those without the diagnosis differ from each other in the same precursors and many concomitants, which may indicate resistance or resilience to the disorder of interest. Which of these are clinically significant only adds to the puzzle.

Thus every DSM categorical diagnosis would be enhanced with a dimensional adjunct, and the challenge to choose the appropriate dimensional diagnosis for each disorder is to identify the most clinically important sources of heterogeneity among those who have the categorical diagnosis and among those who do not. Is it the heterogeneity in severity of symptoms, or is it the impairment induced? Is it the consistency with which symptoms are expressed, or the duration of symptoms? Is it the inability to inhibit symptom expression, lack of control? All of these and more are possibilities that the experts in each disorder must consider.

But perhaps for some DSM categorical diagnoses, adding a dimensional diagnosis might be desirable, but not possible. Current DSM categorical diagnoses are already frequently based on dichotomizing dimensional diagnoses. Consequently, it is difficult to argue that developing dimensional diagnoses cannot be done. Every categorical diagnosis can be made dimensional by using symptom counts, symptom duration, symptom severity, degree of impairment, certainty of diagnosis, consensus of multiple diagnoses, and many more such strategies, even without deviating from the contents of current DSM categorical diagnoses. Thus the issue is not whether a dimensional diagnosis can be added to each categorical diagnosis, it is merely how best to do that for each.

## TWO ILLUSTRATIONS OF IMPACT

### A Thought Experiment

There has long been an extensive literature documenting the advantages of dimensional over categorical measures in research, but the potential impact still seems not well understood. To give a dramatic example, suppose there were a mental health disorder that was caused by a single gene: i.e., if we could get an error-free measure of the expression of that gene, $G^*$, and an error-free dimensional diagnosis of the disorder, $D^*$, the correlation between $G^*$ and $D^*$ would be perfect. The

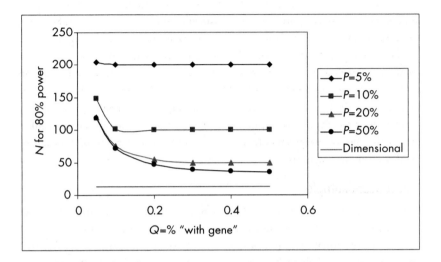

**FIGURE 2–1.** Sample size necessary to achieve 80% power with a 5% one-tailed test to detect a positive correlation between "the gene" and a categorical diagnosis in which the percentage with the diagnosis is *P* and the percentage with "the gene" is *Q*.

Also shown is the sample size necessary if using a dimensional diagnosis.

problem is, of course, we cannot get error-free measures of either. Instead, suppose *G* and *D* are obtainable dimensional measures of $G^*$ and $D^*$ with a validity of, say, 0.6. Then the correlation between *G* and *D* is not 1.0, but 0.6. Whereas it would take a sample size of no more than 10 to detect that perfect correlation between $G^*$ and $D^*$, to achieve 80% power with a 5% one-tailed test to detect positive association between *G* and *D* would require only $N = 13$.

However, suppose now we dichotomized *G*, to represent the presence/absence of the single gene that determined $G^*$, and *D* for a categorical diagnosis. In Figure 2–1 is shown the total sample size necessary to have credibility and adequate power to detect a positive association when the proportion "with the gene" is *Q* and the proportion with a positive diagnosis is *P*. As can be seen, the optimal dichotomization is when both *G* and *D* are dichotomized at their medians, in which case the sample size necessary for 80% power is approximately three times as great as that using dimensional *G* and *D*. When the dichotomization is less than optimal, resulting in small *P* and *Q* as so often happens with diagnoses, the sample size necessary for 80% power may be five or even 10 times as large as that necessary using the dimensional *G* and *D*. In this illustration, we start with perfect correlation and, with unavoidable unreliability of measurement coupled with categorical measures, end with a relation difficult to document as non-random. Moreover, since unreliability and dichotomization both attenuate effect size, the actually perfect correlation between $G^*$ and $D^*$ might in the end be characterized as "small" or, at best, "moderate" and often reported as not statistically significant association. So easy is it to cause even perfect association between a gene and a disorder to disappear.

There is a considerable methodological literature documenting the losses associated with using a categorical variable when a dimensional variable is available (Cohen 1983; Donner and Eliasziw 1994; Kraemer and Thiemann 1987). It is a rare circumstance, likely only in the absence of clinically relevant heterogeneity among those with and without the dichotomous diagnosis, when for purposes of inference in the clinic or in research, there is not a loss of precision and power in using the dichotomous diagnosis.

## A Practical Example

But, some would protest, that could not happen in reality. Theoretical arguments are often not quite as convincing as a real example. Consider then the following: Agras et al. (personal communication, manuscript in preparation) conducted a four-site randomized clinical trial to test the relative effectiveness of cognitive behavior therapy (CBT) against self-help for eating disorders and, more specifically, to test whether a risk classification at entry to the study moderated the effect of CBT versus self-help, as suggested from exploratory studies in earlier randomized clinical trials (Kraemer et al. 2006). In this study, there were 285 subjects distributed over the four sites. The outcome measure, as is typical in this field, was a categorical one, where success was defined as binge frequency and purge frequency below specified cut points, with little or no empirical evidence documenting that the cut points were optimal. No significant treatment effect was found, nor was any significance found for the proposed moderator of treatment. Since nonsignificant effects cannot be interpreted as support for the null hypothesis, the result of this study was a "hung jury."

Suppose instead we were here to use a dimensional measure, the weighted sum of the binge and purge frequencies maximally correlated with the usual categorical outcome (developed using logistic regression with the categorical outcome as the dependent measure and with binge and purge frequencies as the independent measures). If the analysis were done using the dimensional measure (same subjects, same treatments, same design), there is a statistically significant moderator effect of risk strata ($P = 0.023$). Indeed, in the low-risk stratum, CBT was better than self-help with NNT = 9, but in the high-risk stratum the result was in the opposite direction: self-help was better than CBT again with NNT = 9. Such a finding is important since it suggests different choices of treatment for those in the high- and low-risk strata.

What was seen in this study is not unusual. In many of the results of randomized clinical trials or of risk studies that use categorical measures, a report of statistical nonsignificance may be partially or wholly due to the lack of power to detect effects due to use of categorical measures, particularly when the cutoff defining the categorical measures is set by intuition rather than optimally based on empirical evidence. Conversely, the reason sample sizes must be as large as they are (thus taking more time and requiring greater funding investment) may be related to the pervasive use of categorical diagnoses.

## WHAT IF THIS PROPOSAL WERE ACCEPTED? OBJECTIONS

The proposal to include dimensional diagnoses into DSM-V is not without objections, well represented by those of Michael First (2005). First points out the lack of data about clinical utility and user acceptability, and clearly both are important. However, until a dimensional diagnosis is included in a version of DSM, there can be no documentation of either the clinical utility or user acceptability. First (2005) also suggests that inclusion of a dimensional diagnosis will complicate medical record keeping and create administrative and clinical barriers between mental disorders and medical conditions. However, most medical categorical diagnoses already include a dimensional diagnosis as well. When the physician gives a diagnosis of hypertension, the systolic and diastolic blood pressure are recorded; a diagnosis of breast cancer is extended by noting the stage and/or the Karnofsky score; a diagnosis of diabetes, by noting the fasting blood sugar level, etc. First (2005) suggests that inclusion of a dimensional diagnosis in DSM-V would require a massive re-treading effort. Any change in a diagnostic system as established as DSM is always disruptive.

However, mental health providers have long used individually chosen dimensional measures (e.g., the Hamilton score for depression). What inclusion of a dimensional diagnosis in DSM-V would accomplish would be to coordinate the use of dimensional diagnoses across clinicians with the benefits obtained similar to those obtained when the use of categorical diagnoses was coordinated in the earliest DSMs. Similarly, First (2005) suggests that adding a dimensional component might disrupt research efforts, for example, making it impossible to pool studies using DSM-IV and DSM-V. Unfortunately this is true, but it pertains to any change in the categorical diagnoses as well. Any change in the criteria raises issues as to whether research done with one version of DSM can be validly pooled with another version of DSM. Since a dimensional diagnosis in DSM-V would not displace the categorical diagnosis, introduction of a dimensional diagnosis would have less impact in this regard than does any modification of the categorical diagnosis, and there will undoubtedly be such modification. Similarly, First's (2005) concern that inclusion of a dimensional component would complicate clinicians' efforts to integrate prior clinical research using DSM categories into clinical practice applies more to the modification of the categorical diagnosis than it would to an added dimensional diagnosis. Research using the dimensional diagnosis would only begin after DSM-V.

## WHAT IF THIS PROPOSAL WERE ACCEPTED?
## CRITERIA AND CAVEATS

To achieve what is hoped from addition of a dimensional diagnosis into DSM-V, there are certain criteria that would have to be met, and certain approaches may be less than fruitful.

- It is crucial that a DSM-V dimensional diagnosis correspond well with its categorical diagnosis. Those with a positive categorical diagnosis should have dimensional diagnoses much higher than those with a negative categorical diagnosis. Conversely, if one stratifies the population on the dimensional diagnosis, the probability of a positive categorical diagnosis should consistently increase as the dimensional diagnosis increases. If this were not so, research using the categorical and dimensional diagnoses ostensibly for a single disorder would actually deal with two different disorders. It would be difficult, if not impossible, to reconcile the conclusions from studies. With a close positive correlation between the categorical and dimensional diagnoses, the major source of discrepancy between studies done using the two will lie in the greater power and precision of studies using the dimensional diagnosis.
- DSM is meant for the use of clinicians and thus must be transparent to clinicians. Complex algorithms for computation of a dimensional diagnosis will not be useful to clinicians, and research based on such diagnoses will not be easily interpretable by clinicians. Consider the Framingham Index, a dimensional measure indicating risk for cardiac events (Truett et al. 1967). This index requires, for example, that the clinician assess the patient's age, gender, smoking status, and whether or not the patient is on medication for high blood pressure, total cholesterol, high-density lipoprotein cholesterol, or systolic blood pressure. From this information a weighted score is computed from which the probability of a future cardiac event can be estimated. Score sheets are available and calculators appear on the Web, but the calculation of such a risk score has not become a routine procedure for clinicians. However, a simplified version in which each of the indicators is dichotomized and given a point count indicating the importance of each indicator, with the total point count convertible to a risk level, is also available. This simplified version of a dimensional score may not be as accurate a predictor of cardiac risk, but because the clinician can see exactly what goes into the score and needs no complex computation procedure, it is more likely to be used in practice. In the same way, every effort should be made to make the DSM-V dimensional diagnosis clinically useful, if not necessarily mathematically elegant. Consequently, there are certain paths to the development of dimensional diagnosis that must be viewed with concern. While completely subjective and non-evidence-based decision-making is likely to subvert the process, complex mathematical models, based on assumptions that

may or may not be true, may generate dimensional diagnoses not only non-transparent to clinicians, but very possibly nonvalid. At the other extreme, complex mathematical methods (latent variable modeling, item response theory, etc.) are valuable tools to be used to help generate possible approaches to dimensional diagnoses, but if what results does not correspond to clinical knowledge and insight, and is not verified for test–retest reliability and validity against external criteria, these results may also subvert efforts.

• Finally, the dimensional diagnosis, as is also true of the categorical diagnosis, must show good test–retest reliability, have clinical validity, and withstand more demanding challenges to validity. Consequently, the dimensional diagnosis, as is also true of the categorical diagnosis, must be evidence-based, reflecting what has been learned about diagnosis in the years since the introduction of DSM-IV. The emphasis in the evidence must be on effect sizes, which indicate clinical significance, and not on statistical significance ($P$ values), for all the reasons made ever clearer in recent years of the limitations of statistical hypothesis testing when the focus is on $P$ values rather than effect sizes (Borenstein 1997; Cohen 1995; Dar et al. 1994; Hunter 1997; Jacobson and Truax 1991; Kraemer 1993; Kraemer et al. 1999; Schmidt 1996; Shrout 1997; Thompson 1999; Wilkinson 1999).

## Discussion and Conclusions

The discussion about adding a dimensional component to DSM has been ongoing for many years. In the earliest stages of development of each version of DSM since DSM-III, the idea has surfaced and then again submerged. The time to include a dimensional diagnosis is now, with DSM-V, not only because the arguments for doing so are so strong but also to begin to prepare for the possible inclusion of genetic, imaging, biochemical, or other signals into future diagnostic systems.

The process of adding a dimensional component to DSM at this time can be made as simple or as complicated as is appropriate given the state of knowledge about each disorder. Personality disorders, for example, have long focused on dimensional diagnosis and are likely more than ready to move in this direction. Other diagnoses have given the idea and process less thought, and may be at an earlier phase of the process. The first version of a dimensional diagnosis, like the earliest versions of categorical diagnoses, is unlikely to be anywhere near perfect. However, as dimensional diagnosis is proposed, used, and evaluated, it too, like categorical diagnosis, will improve with time and the accrual of evidence based on those diagnoses.

Nevertheless, the consequences of including a dimensional component in DSM-V may revolutionize psychiatric research and clinical decision-making, and bring progress in dealing with mental disorders more in line with progress in dealing with other medical conditions.

# References

American Psychiatric Association. Diagnostic and Statistical Manual: Mental Disorders. Washington, DC: American Psychiatric Association, 1952.

American Psychiatric Association. Diagnostic and Statistical Manual of Mental Disorders, 2nd Edition. Washington, DC: American Psychiatric Association, 1968.

American Psychiatric Association. Diagnostic and Statistical Manual of Mental Disorders, 3rd Edition. Washington, DC: American Psychiatric Association, 1980.

American Psychiatric Association. Diagnostic and Statistical Manual of Mental Disorders, 4th Edition. Washington, DC: American Psychiatric Association, 1994.

Borenstein M. Hypothesis testing and effect size estimation in clinical trials. Ann Allergy Asthma Immunol 1997; 78: 5–16.

Caplan PJ. They say you're crazy: how the world's most powerful psychiatrists decide who's normal. Cambridge, MA: Da Capo Press, 1995.

Cohen J. The cost of dichotomization. Applied Psychological Measurement 1983; 7(3): 249–253.

Cohen J. The Earth is round ($p < 0.05$). Am Psychol 1995; 49: 997–1003.

Dar R, Serlin RC, Omer H. Misuse of statistical tests in three decades of psychotherapy research. J Consult Clin Psychol 1994; 62: 75–82.

Donner A, Eliasziw M. Statistical implications of the choice between a dichotomous or continuous trait in studies of interobserver agreement. Biometrics 1994; 50: 550–555.

First MB. Clinical utility: a prerequisite for the adoption of a dimensional approach in DSM. J Abnorm Psychol 2005; 114(4): 560–564.

Hunter JE. Needed: a ban on the significance test. Psychol Sci 1997; 8(1): 3–7.

Jacobson NS, Truax P. Clinical significance: a statistical approach to defining meaningful change in psychotherapy research. J Consul Clin Psychol 1991; 59(1): 12–19.

Kirk SA, Kutchins H. The Selling of the DSM: The Rhetoric of Science in Psychiatry. New York: Aldine de Gruyter, 1992.

Kraemer HC. To increase power in randomized clinical trials without increasing sample size. Psychopharmacol Bull 1991; 27(3): 217–224.

Kraemer HC. Reporting the size of effects in research studies to facilitate assessment of practical or clinical significance. Psychoneuroendocrinology 1993; 17: 527–536.

Kraemer HC, O'Hara R. Categorical versus dimensional approaches to diagnosis: methodological challenges. J Psychiatr Res 2004; 38(1): 17–25.

Kraemer HC, Thiemann S. How Many Subjects? Statistical Power Analysis in Research. Newbury Park, CA: Sage Publications, 1987.

Kraemer HC, Thiemann SA. A strategy to use soft data effectively in randomized clinical trials. J Consult Clin Psychol 1989; 57: 148–154.

Kraemer HC, Kazdin AE, Offord DR, Kessler RC, Jensen PS, Kupfer DJ. Measuring the potency of a risk factor for clinical or policy significance. Psychol Methods 1999; 4(3): 257–271.

Kraemer HC, Periyakoil VS, Noda A. Tutorial in biostatistics: kappa coefficients in medical research. Stat Med 2002; 21: 2109–2129.

Kraemer HC, Frank E, Kupfer DJ. Moderators of treatment outcomes: clinical, research, and policy importance. JAMA 2006; 296(10): 1–4.

Kupfer DJ, Thase ME. Laboratory studies and validity of psychiatric diagnosis: has there been progress? In Robbins LN, Barrett JE (eds) The Validity of Psychiatric Diagnosis. New York: Raven Press, 1989, pp. 177–201.

Lord FM, Novick MR. Statistical Theories of Mental Test Scores. Reading, MA: Addison-Wesley Publishing Company, 1968.

Robins E, Guze SB. Establishment of diagnostic validity in psychiatric illness: its application to schizophrenia. Am J Psychiatry 1970; 126: 983–987.

Robins LN, Barrett JE (eds). The Validity of Psychiatric Diagnosis. New York: Raven Press, 1989.

Schmidt FL. Statistical significance testing and cumulative knowledge in psychology: implications for training of researchers. Psychol Methods 1996; 1(2): 115–129.

Shrout PE. Should significance tests be banned? introduction to a special section exploring the pros and cons. Psychol Sci 1997; 8(1): 1–2.

Thompson B. Journal editorial policies regarding statistical significance tests: heat is to fire as p is to importance. Educational Psychology Review 1999; 11: 157–169.

Truett J, Cornfield J, Kannel WA. A multivariate analysis of the risk of coronary heart disease in Framingham. J Chronic Dis 1967; 20: 511–524.

Wilkinson L. Task Force on Statistical Inference. Statistical methods in psychology journals: guidelines and explanations. Am Psychol 1999; 54: 594–604.

# 3

# A DIMENSIONAL OPTION FOR THE DIAGNOSIS OF SUBSTANCE DEPENDENCE IN DSM-V

John E. Helzer, M.D.
Kathleen K. Bucholz, Ph.D.
Michael Gossop, Ph.D.

In this chapter we offer a model for creating dimensional diagnoses for the *Diagnostic and Statistical Manual of Mental Disorders,* Fifth Edition (DSM-V) substance use disorders (SUDs) in a way that can be related back to their corresponding categorical definitions. For illustration, we use the existing DSM-IV (American Psychiatric Association 1994) definition for the alcohol use disorders (AUDs) as the prototype and discuss the application of such a prototype to all of the SUDs. We begin the chapter with a review of empirical evidence regarding the dimensionality

Reprinted with permission from Helzer JE, Bucholz KK, Gossop M. "A Dimensional Option for the Diagnosis of Substance Dependence in DSM-IV." *International Journal of Methods in Psychiatric Research* 2007; 16(S1): S24–S33.

This work was supported by the following grants: AA11954, AA14270, AA015777 (JEH), AA11667, AA12640, AA11998, U10AA08401, and DA14363 (KKB). The authors would also like to acknowledge Dr. Wilson Compton, Director, Division of Epidemiology, Services and Prevention Research at NIDA for his assistance in conceptualizing the issues discussed in this chapter and for reading and commenting on the manuscript.

of SUDs, focusing primarily on diagnoses of dependence. The abuse diagnosis applies to certain substances and not others (e.g., tobacco) and is a more contentious construct, as indicated by the fact that the two major nosological systems, DSM and *International Classification of Diseases* (ICD), do not agree. However, there is growing evidence that the DSM-V symptoms of abuse and dependence may form a single continuum, at least for some substances. Where problems of abuse and dependence have been considered together, we address the evidence accordingly.

# Literature Review

## ALCOHOL

The rudiments of dimensionality in the AUDs may be seen in Jellinek's (1960) developmental stages of alcoholism and are firmly embedded in the work of Edwards and Gross (1976; Edwards 1977, 1986), where dimensionality of the alcohol dependence syndrome (ADS) is reflected not only in two proposed axes, dependence and alcohol-related disabilities, but also in the conceptualization of the syndrome itself as occurring "with graded intensity" (Edwards 1977). Skinner and colleagues, in a series of empirical analyses largely based on clinical samples, proposed a hybrid conceptualization of the ADS that combined subtypes (categories) that were ordered along a dimension reflecting the "global severity of the symptoms of alcohol dependence" (Morey and Skinner 1986; Morey et al. 1984).

In 1987, DSM, long considered a proponent of categorical diagnoses, acknowledged that mental disorders should not be assumed to be sharply bounded discrete entities. The shift in diagnostic criteria from DSM-III (American Psychiatric Association 1980), where specific symptoms were required, to DSM-III-R (American Psychiatric Association 1987), where a certain number of symptoms were needed, presaged dimensionality, at least with respect to SUDs. Options for coding diagnoses as "mild," "moderate," or "severe" were made explicit in SUD criteria in DSM-III-R. In DSM-IV, more attention was given to dimensionalizing disorders, particularly for "describing phenomena that are distributed continuously and that do not have clear boundaries" (p. xxii). Still, it was noted that these minor efforts had been "less useful than categorical systems in clinical practice and in stimulating research," although "increasing research on…dimensional systems may eventually result in their greater acceptance both as a method of conveying clinical information and as a research tool" (p. xxii). It is fair to say that, at least with respect to SUDs, we are at that point envisioned in 1994.

There is now a plethora of studies from which evidence for a unidimensional construct of alcohol dependence has evolved. From early descriptive studies (Rohan 1976), methodology graduated to factor analysis of 11 symptoms of abuse and dependence and evidence of a single-factor solution (Hall et al. 1993; Hasin et al. 1994; Proudfoot et al. 2006). A series of latent class analyses of 37 alcohol abuse and dependence symptoms reported by middle-aged male twins in Australia (Heath et al. 1994), 38 alcohol abuse/dependence symptom data reported by relatives of alcoholic probands in the Collaborative Study on the Genetics of Alcoholism (Bucholz et al. 1996), and 11 items of abuse and dependence from young adult male and female twins from the Australian Twin Register (Lynskey et al. 2005) reach the same conclusion: that symptoms were arrayed on a continuum of severity rather than in unique categories. There are also some reports of factor analytic studies resulting in two-factor solutions (e.g., Harford and Muthen 2001; Muthen 1995, 1996; Muthen et al. 1993a, 1993b; Nelson et al. 1999). However, these findings may be less discrepant than they appear since correlations between the factors in some studies where two-factor solutions were selected are quite high, suggesting a one-factor solution might actually have been preferable.

Other investigators have applied item response theory (IRT) to data on symptoms of alcohol dependence and abuse from a variety of samples. Inferences have been remarkably consistent that alcohol symptoms of DSM-IV dependence and abuse are unidimensional and arrayed along a continuum of severity. This conclusion holds across a variety of samples, including fathers of adolescent-aged twins (Krueger et al. 2004), college students (Kahler et al. 2004), adult patients in treatment for alcoholism (Kahler et al. 2003; Langenbucher et al. 2004), current (Saha et al. 2006) and lifetime (Kahler and Strong 2006) drinkers from a national probability sample of adults in the United States, and adolescents in treatment for AUD (Martin et al. 2006). Illustrative of this line of research, Saha et al. (2006) analyzed the 11 alcohol abuse and dependence criteria from DSM-IV for the past 12 months from reports of 22,526 current drinkers in the National Epidemiologic Survey on Alcohol and Related Conditions (NESARC) study (Grant et al. 2003, 2004). They found that the symptoms (with the exception of legal problems due to drinking) reflected a continuum of severity. No clear distinction between abuse and dependence symptoms was observed. They also suggested that the DSM-IV items captured the severe end of the spectrum but overlooked the mild to moderate range. However, in a second paper, Saha et al. (2007) found that a standard measure of consumption (five or more drinks in one drinking occasion for men, four or more for women) at least once a week in the past year fit well into the same dimensional continuum described in their previous paper and could be used as a marker for the mild to moderate end of the continuum. Kahler and Strong (2006), using 33 individual lifetime symptoms of alcohol abuse and dependence in the NESARC sample, also reached the conclusion that alcohol abuse and dependence symptoms were unidimensional. Like Saha et al. (2006), they observed some abuse items manifesting greater severity than some dependence symptoms, blurring the distinction between the two. In yet another application of IRT methods to 11 lifetime criteria of DSM-IV alcohol abuse and dependence in a treatment sample of adolescents, Martin et al. (2006) observed a unidimensional trait of severity of alcohol problems, and greater severity of certain abuse symptoms over some dependence items. Collectively, these studies provide good evidence of the unidimensionality of alcohol items.

Recently, an analysis of two large probability general population samples of adults in the United States that avoids making the strong assumptions inherent in IRT or latent class analysis provided further support for a dimensional configuration for alcohol dependence (Hasin et al. 2006). Testing five alternatives of DSM-IV alcohol dependence criteria (reflecting categorical, dimensional, and hybrid versions of alcohol dependence) with three validating variables (family history, treatment, and early onset), the authors found that a model formulating alcohol dependence criteria as a one-dimensional linear predictor optimally explained the relationships with the three validators. The authors concluded that, while categorical diagnoses serve important clinical purposes, inclusion of a dimensional indicator of alcohol dependence would enhance and promote research objectives.

## SUBSTANCES OTHER THAN ALCOHOL

In the smaller body of work exploring dependence on substances other than alcohol, samples are less diverse, and statistical techniques less sophisticated. Nevertheless, the available evidence supports the unidimensionality of the dependence construct in other substances as well. Coverage is uneven, with cocaine, opiates, and cannabis among those most commonly studied. In clinical and mixed samples, researchers have found evidence for unidimensionality of the dependence construct for cannabis (Feingold and Rounsaville 1995; Langenbucher et al. 2004; Martin et al. 2006; Morgenstern et al. 1994), opiates (Feingold and Rounsaville 1995; Gossop et al. 1995; Hasin et al. 1988; Kosten et al. 1987; Morgenstern et al. 1994), cocaine (Feingold and Rounsaville 1995; Gossop et al. 1995; Hasin et al. 1988; Kosten et al. 1987; Langenbucher et al. 2004; Morgenstern et al. 1994), amphetamines (Feingold and Rounsaville 1995; Gossop et al. 1995; Hasin et al. 1988; Morgenstern et al. 1994), and sedatives (Feingold and Rounsaville 1995; Hasin et al. 1988; Morgenstern et al. 1994).

Gossop et al. (1995), in a sample of 1,312 users of opiates, cocaine, and amphetamines recruited from clinical and non-clinical settings, found strong evidence for unidimensionality using the Severity of Dependence Scale for all three substances in principal components factor analyses. All analyses revealed a single-factor solution; validity was supported by high correlations with variables reflecting severity of disorder. Single-factor solutions for cocaine and opiates have been reported by Kosten et al. (1987) in a sample of psychiatric inpatients. Morgenstern et al. (1994), in their factor analysis of data from adults in treatment for alcohol or drug problems, observed that one factor captured dependence criteria for cannabis, cocaine, stimulants, sedatives, and opiates. In data from a sample of inpatients in an alcohol rehabilitation unit, Hasin et al. (1988) reported a single factor underlying dependence for cocaine, stimulants, sedatives, opiates, and hallucinogens. Feingold and Rounsaville (1995), using data from both clinical and community subjects, applied confirmatory factor analysis and also found a single factor for dependence for cocaine, cannabis, opiates, sedatives, and stimulants. Teesson et al. (2002), applying confirmatory factor analysis to data from the Australian general population, reported that a single-factor model was the best-fitting solution.

Applying IRT to data on 11 dependence and abuse items for cocaine, cannabis, and alcohol obtained from adults in treatment, Langenbucher et al. (2004) found that a unidimensional model fit the data for cocaine, but only fit those for alcohol and cannabis when two items were removed (one from abuse, one from dependence). In one of the few studies of adolescents in treatment, Martin et al. (2006) obtained good fit to a model reflecting a single dimension of problem severity for both alcohol and cannabis. Kirisci et al. (2002) also observed a single unidimensional trait in their IRT analysis of men from clinical and volunteer samples, in female spouses of drug-dependent men, and in offspring of men with SUD (Kirisci et al. 2006).

Several studies have challenged the interpretation of one dimension for dependence, including Morgenstern et al. (1994) for hallucinogen dependence, Bryant et al. (1991) for cocaine dependence, and Kosten et al. (1987) for sedatives, cannabis, hallucinogens, and sedatives. Nelson et al. (1999), using data from community and treatment multicultural samples, found that while the evidence supported a single underlying factor for cannabis, cocaine, and opiates overall, this finding did not hold for low to moderate users, which led them to suggest that studies based on homogeneous samples (such as clinical samples) may be biased towards selecting lesser-order solutions. Clearly, additional analyses of the currently available large general population data sets are in order.

## TOBACCO

Although there is a paucity of studies examining the dimensionality of tobacco dependence criteria, findings from most of them indicate that, unlike other substances, tobacco dependence is not unidimensional. Johnson et al. (1996) found two factors in a sample of young adult daily smokers; Muthen and Asparouhov (2006) in a general population sample selected multiple-factor models over a single-factor model; Hughes et al. (2004) reached that same conclusion, as did Radzius et al. (2004) who identified, in a sample of cigarette smokers who were volunteers, the same two factors identified by Johnson et al. (1996). A study that has reported unidimensional results (Strong et al. 2003) used a modeling procedure with very strong assumptions, analyzed lifetime symptoms, and did not have all dependence items available. Thus, among the few studies that exist, the weight of evidence does not support unidimensionality. Instead, it suggests that tobacco dependence represents a potential anomaly within the current DSM-IV diagnostic system that poses a challenge both to generic approaches to diagnosis and to attempts to construct a generic dimensional measure of dependence. Many nicotine researchers do not use the DSM/ICD system, choosing instead to use scales that do not encompass DSM/ICD criteria (Hughes et al. 2004). Reconciling this contrast could be a challenge to the DSM-V Substance Use Disorders Workgroup and thus should be a part of a research agenda in preparation for the revision process.

## SUMMARY OF THE LITERATURE

Overall, our review of the literature indicates that for both AUDs and for most substances other than alcohol, dimensionality of the dependence construct is well established. Tobacco dependence is a possible exception to this generalization. Future research should focus on applying the rigorous statistical techniques observed for AUDs to substances other than alcohol, including tobacco.

# Potential Advantages, Drawbacks, and Challenges for a Dimensional Approach

A dimensional option for the assessment of the SUDs is consistent both with current knowledge and practice. A good deal of evidence specifically regards the dependence syndrome as a dimensional construct. A standardized rating system for individual symptoms would contribute to knowledge of the nature and severity of the symptomatic components of the dependence syndrome. Clinicians and researchers would benefit from a quantitative assessment of severity in addition to presence/absence of a diagnostic entity; the use of quantitative measurements avoids the loss of information associated with a categorical assessment.

Clinical decisions often require categorical judgments. However, different categorical cutoff points may lead to differing or even opposite clinical conclusions. In clinical practice, a dimensional measure of dependence would not replace but would supplement the categorical diagnosis. A quantitative measure avoids the problems that arise with any strict categorical cutoff (e.g., borderline cases). Most studies that have supported the dimensional construct of dependence have not found evidence of a specific categorical cutoff that clearly differentiates cases from non-cases.

A dimensional measure of severity can serve as a moderator variable that affects treatment outcome. For example, dimensional measures of opiate dependence and alcohol dependence act independently as moderators of substance use outcomes in the treatment of illicit drug misusers (Gossop et al. 2006). A trial comparing naltrexone and acamprosate in the treatment of alcohol dependence showed no overall difference between the two treatments (Morley et al. 2006). However, the inclusion of a dimensional measure of dependence showed differential outcomes for patients with low levels of alcohol dependence versus patients with higher levels.

A dimensional approach is also consistent with recent neurobiological research into the cellular activity and neural circuitry of addiction. The concept of addiction as a developmental process that may be found in varying degrees of severity is supported by the findings that cellular changes in prefrontal glutamatergic activity of the accumbens play an important role in determining the compulsive behaviors of the addictions by reducing the impact of natural rewards, diminishing cognitive control, and increasing responsiveness to drug-related stimuli (Kalivas and Volkow 2005).

Few drug takers use only a single substance, and polysubstance use complicates the assessment and diagnostic process. A dimensional assessment can provide separate scores across substances to identify those most in need of treatment. Adding dimensional scores across substances offers a single measure for total substance involvement and could provide a basis for further research investigation into the additive, interactive, or other relationship that may exist in relation to dependence upon more than one substance. Obviously, for dimensions to be additive across substances, the scales must be created for each substance in the same way. The methodology we propose later for scale creation is indeed applicable for all substances, with the possible exception of tobacco.

A similar problem arises with co-occurring psychiatric disorders and SUDs. A dimensional system of assessment permits separate severity scores to be allocated to each syndrome and provides patient-specific quantitative profiles. Dimensional assessments can be used whether or not each syndrome meets the threshold for a categorical diagnosis. A dimensional system may, therefore, provide a more complete assessment of the patient's comorbidity, thus facilitating appropriate treatment.

A dimensional assessment within the DSM system would encourage the wider use of quantitative measurement of dependence in the broader field of addiction studies. A quantitative dimensional measure would also support a more uniform approach. Rather than the inconsistency associated with choosing among the several dimensional scales that are already available, a standardized DSM dimensional approach would promote consistency and improve cross-study comparability. Although the utility of a categorical diagnosis within clinical contexts is a priority, a dimensional approach would be more useful than a categorical system for research with non-clinical samples. For example, a dimensional assessment of dependence would have greater relevance and applicability in public health and epidemiological studies, where categorical diagnoses can be problematic. Most positive cases cluster at the categorical diagnostic threshold (Helzer et al. 1985), thus even a slight degree of error variance can result in considerable diagnostic instability.

# Remaining Questions for a Research Agenda

There could be concern about how a standardized dimensional assessment of dependence would be affected by its application in languages other than English or in cultures other than North America. However, instruments that provide dimensional measures of dependence have been successfully used across languages and cultures. The Severity of Dependence Scale, for example, has been used in many other languages, including Russian, Chinese, Spanish, Portuguese, Polish, Czech, Farsi, Indonesian, and Thai (World Health Organization 2006). In another World Health Organization project (Hall et al. 1993), Alcohol Use Disorders Identification Test (AUDIT) data from six different countries were analyzed by principal-component analyses. The results showed a strong general factor, supporting the suggestion that the alcohol dependence syndrome has cross-cultural generalizability. However, there were differences between countries, with some respondents (in India) appearing to have difficulty understanding the constructs underlying the questions. Further study is required of effects of sociocultural and linguistic differences upon dimensional measures of dependence. Given the international impact of DSM, a consistent approach within the classification would encourage such exploration. It is also straightforward to norm a dimensional scale for each population.

Another topic for a research agenda is the optimum design of an SUD dimensional scale. A consideration of advantages and disadvantages cannot be accomplished simply by means of a list; many options will be both advantageous in some respects but disadvantageous in others. A complex scale may confer benefits in terms of mathematical properties and consequent statistical power. But this may be achieved at the cost of greater difficulties for the respondent and scale administrator in terms of user-friendliness, comprehension, or response burden. Whatever dimensional system is adopted, it should be easily understood and readily usable in a clinical setting. Its relationship to the categorical criteria should be understandable. Its use should also be optional for clinicians and investigators, not a requirement for a DSM diagnosis. In the next section we propose a model for a dimensional scale that meets these criteria.

Despite many similarities between different dependence disorders, further consideration must be given to the pros and cons of generic versus drug-specific criteria for dependence. In particular, issues need to be resolved regarding item weighting. It cannot be assumed that all items have equal significance, nor that they have the same significance for different substances. Some symptoms may be more important than others in quantifying the diagnosis. For instance, there is broad agreement that a primary behavioral pathology in drug addiction is the overpowering motivational strength and decreased ability to control the desire to obtain drugs (Kalivas and Volkow 2005). However, the construction of appropriately weighted dependence items is a complex task. This is further complicated when these are applied to different substances and across a variety of countries. Dimensional assessments of dependence may have different diagnostic implications for different substances. Dependence upon some substances is associated with a clinically important withdrawal syndrome. For other substances, the presence of a withdrawal syndrome is less clear and may be of less clinical significance.

As noted earlier, nicotine dependence represents a potential anomaly within the current DSM-IV diagnostic system. Nicotine dependence poses a challenge to generic approaches to diagnosis and to attempts to construct a generic dimensional measure of dependence. Most nicotine dependence scales do not include DSM/ICD criteria. Many nicotine researchers do not make use of the current DSM or ICD systems.

# Specific Proposal for a Substance Use Disorders Dimensional Option for DSM-V

It is clear from the earlier review and discussion that incorporating a dimensional approach could enhance both clinical and research utility of the DSM-V SUDs. However, any such addition must be done in a way that preserves the traditional, categorical approach of the DSM. Categorical and dimensional approaches offer differing but equally important taxonomic functions (Kraemer 2007). In this section we propose a model for adding dimensional components that are based upon the categorical illness definitions in DSM-V.

## STEP ONE: DEFINING CATEGORIES

Our proposal for adding dimensions to DSM begins with the DSM-V diagnostic workgroups creating categorical illness definitions, just as they have in the previous revisions of DSM. As before, this includes deciding what signs and symptoms to include in each category and what the categorical threshold should be for each diagnosis. If a dimensional option is based on that categorical definition, it will ensure concordance between the two approaches, which is far preferable to two independent sets of criteria.

The substance category could include definitions for both abuse and dependence if the workgroup so chooses, but it would be highly advantageous if the workgroup was cognizant of findings from the published literature cited earlier on the dimensional pattern of symptoms, so that symptoms at the mild end of the substance continuum could be designated in the abuse category and symptoms that fall at the more severe end could be included in dependence. Further, if the weekly 5+/4+ consumption criterion proposed by Saha et al. (2007) were added to the categorical definition, it would appear to strengthen the mild-to-moderate range of the dimensional definition. These considerations would help to ensure a single, broadly encompassing dimension for the SUDs even if there are separate categorical distinctions for abuse and dependence.

## STEP TWO: DIMENSIONALIZING SYMPTOMS

After the symptoms for a particular diagnosis have been defined by the diagnostic workgroup(s), the next step would be to create a dimensional scale for each symptom. This could be done using a simple scale that is uniform across symptoms and across the substance diagnoses or by using a more complex scale that is symptom- and/or diagnosis-specific. A simple, uniform method might be to score each symptom on a three-point scale logically based on symptom severity or frequency, whichever is more appropriate. For example, substance withdrawal might logically be scored in terms of severity: none (never occurred), mild (has occurred but never severe), or severe. However, a symptom such as sacrificing other activities in order to use a substance might be more logically scored in terms of its frequency of occurrence: never, sometimes, frequent. In either case, these three levels could correspond to a simple numerical score of 0, 1, or 2. Dimensionalization of individual symptoms could also be done using more complex scales that allow more latitude in the scoring and/or accommodate biological or laboratory measures should they become relevant.

For DSM-V, we would advocate for a simple scoring method. The major disadvantage of a more complex method of dimensionalizing individual symptoms is that it might rapidly become cumbersome, with symptoms across substances, or even within a single substance, being dimensionalized differently. Such an approach might capture more of the relevant dimensional variability, but it would also be much harder to remember, apply, and communicate. The dimensional scale for a diagnosis could in effect become a black box rather than a more transparent and memorable coding applied uniformly across all symptoms and diagnoses. Any final decision about this rests in the hands of the DSM-V Task Force and the individual diagnostic workgroups. But the recommendation of the authors of this chapter would be to opt for a simple, transparent, and easily comprehensible approach at this point in time.

## STEP THREE: CREATING DIMENSIONAL SCALES

Next we propose that the scores for individual symptoms be used collectively to create a quantitative measure for the specific diagnosis. There are a variety of statistical methods available to accomplish this step, such as factor analysis (Muthen et al. 1993a), latent trait modeling (Krueger et al. 2004), IRT (Saha et al. 2006), latent transition analysis (Lanza et al. 2003), or newer methods such as latent class factor analysis, proposed by Muthen and Asparouhov (2006), as appropriate for both categories and dimensions. The relationship between the categorical and the dimensional approaches would depend in large measure on the statistical method chosen for this step. Recommendation of a particular method requires statistical consultation and is beyond the scope of this chapter. This question should be part of the ongoing research agenda and expert discussion in the preparation of DSM-V.

Any of the earlier statistical methods are more appropriate for creating a quantitative diagnostic scale than simply summing the symptom scores. However, no statistical method would result in an interval scale at either the symptom or the diagnostic level. There is no guarantee, for example, that a diagnostic scale score of 6 would represent twice the level of severity as a score of 3. But any of the earlier approaches can be used to create an ordinal scale, the statistical and clinical advantages of which are superior to those of the purely nominal system that DSM has exemplified up to this point in its history.

## STEP FOUR: RELATING SCALES TO CATEGORIES

Once a scale based on dimensionalized symptoms has been created, receiver operating characteristic (ROC) curve analysis (Kraemer et al. 2004) can be used to identify the quantitative score that most closely correlates with the categorical diagnostic threshold originally established by the diagnostic workgroup. This is a particularly important step. As we discussed in the opening section, diagnostic quantification of the SUDs has advantages for both clinical and research uses. An estimate of the score that best relates to the categorical diagnosis helps orient clinicians and investigators, and helps ensure concordance between the categorical and dimensional options. If the workgroup decides that two categorical levels are necessary (e.g., abuse and dependence), it may still be desirable that there be a single dimensional scale. Separate dimensional scales for abuse and dependence would be awkward. However, ROC curve analysis can be used to identify the quantitative score that most closely correlates with each of these categories.

## STRUCTURAL RECOMMENDATIONS

We recommend that a dimensional component for the DSM-V SUDs be based upon the categorical substance definitions that will be created by the Substance-Related Disorders Workgroup. We consider it vital that the categorical and dimensional diagnostic definitions be closely linked. It would serve no one's interest to create separate sets of categorical and dimensional criteria that are independent of one another. The final product of such an approach might conceivably be more psychometrically cohesive than a dimension that is tied to a previously defined categorical definition. But unless the categorical and dimensional are clearly related, it seems likely that diagnostic cacophony would result.

We also strongly recommend that the dimensional approach be an integral part of DSM rather than included as a supplement or an appendix, neither of which is likely to have status or visibility equal to that of the categorical criteria. It seems unequivocal that DSM dimensional criteria would serve the needs of both clinicians and investigators, just as the categorical criteria have since the advent of DSM-III. Once a categorical diagnosis has been made, as clinicians we think in dimensional terms about severity, treatment, and outcome. For the investigator, a dimensional approach adds considerably to the statistical power, permitting a stronger test of scientific hypotheses with smaller sample sizes. In addition, a dimensional scale permits creation of population norms that are sensitive to gender, ethnicity, developmental stage, and culture. For example, in the SUDs, what is deviant in a restrictive culture may not be so in a more permissive one, and what is normal for middle-aged males may not be so for young adolescents. A dimensional scale offers the opportunity of denoting norms and standard deviations for whatever group is being examined in a way that is much more specific than is the case with a categorical definition that must be applied equally to all population groups. Equal status for the categorical and dimensional approaches within the taxonomy helps ensure that full advantage will be taken of the strengths they each have to offer.

## Conclusions

The evidence for offering a dimensional diagnostic option for the diagnosis of substance dependence in DSM-V seems irrefutable. The supportive literature for AUDs is extensive and nearly uniform in suggesting that the signs and symptoms typically considered salient to a categorical diagnosis form a single severity dimension and one that is strongly predictive of outcome. While less extensive and varied, the literature for most other substances included in prior versions of DSM is similarly supportive of a quantitative construct that is likely unidimensional. The conclusion of the authors of this chapter is that the body of empirical evidence cannot be ignored in revising DSM.

In addition to the consistent evidence of a severity continuum detailed earlier, there are other reasons to support the addition of a dimensional diagnostic option for the SUDs. A dimensional approach captures more of the known phenotypic variability that is the key rationale for a taxonomy in the first place. Dimensions help resolve problems of threshold cases and are of greater relevance to studies of longitudinal course, treatment predictions, and comorbidity. Finally, a dimensional option added to categorical diagnoses represents a major taxonomic advance, not a repetition.

Any change in so basic a scientific tool as a diagnostic taxonomy is disruptive. Even revising categorical definitions, as will be done in DSM-V, means that clinical thinking has to be readjusted and that research using prior definitions must be reinterpreted in light of new definitions. Thus it is important that changes in the taxonomy be gradual and evolutionary rather than revolutionary. Regardless of what might evolve in terms of dimensional diagnoses in DSM-V, there is an ongoing need for categorical illness definitions for both clinical and research purposes. Categorical diagnoses are a verbal shorthand facilitating communication between clinicians, between investigators, and between psychiatric professionals and patients. Potential difficulty occurs when we reify the definitions and assume, as we often do, that because two patients fall into the same diagnostic category they are alike in all important respects vis-à-vis that psychiatric illness. But many, if not most, disorders are on a continuum: those falling above a categorical diagnostic threshold differ in severity; those below the threshold vary in how close to the threshold they are. Thus when we design a treatment study of alcohol dependence and analyze the data as if the diagnosis defines a homogeneous group, we sacrifice considerable statistical power by failing to recognize the substantial clinical variability embedded within that categorical label. Nevertheless, the convention of a single diagnostic label for those who share the requisite clinical characteristics in common is both parsimonious and utilitarian and should be preserved.

However, once a categorical diagnosis has been made, a series of quantitative questions arise: Is the illness severe enough that treatment is warranted? How aggressively should I treat? Should immediate hospitalization be considered? As clinicians we grapple with these issues by consulting our own prior experience, but we all tend to do it differently. A defined quantitative scale offers greater consistency in grappling with these quantitative issues, better enabling us to benefit from our own experience, that of our colleagues, and the accumulated research evidence. On the investigative side, scientific progress in psychiatric genetics, genetic epidemiology, imaging, and multiple other areas requiring refinement of diagnostic phenotypes is accelerating. Our taxonomy must keep pace if it is to remain relevant.

Adding a dimensional option to DSM-V while retaining traditional categorical definitions is an evolutionary change that has advantages for clinicians, investigators, and ultimately the entire field of psychiatry. Basing the addition of a dimensional option on the categorical definitions created by the Substance-Related Disorders Workgroup, as we propose here, minimizes any disruption to diagnostic traditions that have proven value.

# References

American Psychiatric Association. Diagnostic and Statistical Manual of Mental Disorders, 3rd Edition. Washington, DC: American Psychiatric Association, 1980.

American Psychiatric Association. Diagnostic and Statistical Manual of Mental Disorders, 3rd Edition, Revised. Washington, DC: American Psychiatric Association, 1987.

American Psychiatric Association. Diagnostic and Statistical Manual of Mental Disorders, 4th Edition. Washington, DC: American Psychiatric Association, 1994.

Bryant KJ, Rounsaville BJ, Babor TF. Coherence of the dependence syndrome in cocaine users. Br J Addict 1991; 86: 1299–1310.

Bucholz KK, Heath AC, Reich T, Hesselbrock VM, Kramer JR, Nurnberger JI Jr, Schuckit MA. Can we subtype alcoholism? a latent class analysis of data from relatives of alcoholics in a multicenter family study of alcoholism. Alcohol Clin Exp Res 1996; 20: 1462–1471.

Edwards G. The alcohol dependence syndrome: usefulness of an idea. In G Edwards, M Grant (eds) Alcoholism, Medicine, and Psychiatry: New Knowledge and New Responses. London: Croom Helm, 1977, pp. 136–156.

Edwards G. The alcohol dependence syndrome: a concept as stimulus to enquiry. Br J Addict 1986; 81: 171–183.

Edwards G, Gross MM. Alcohol dependence: provisional description of a clinical syndrome. Br Med J 1976; 1: 1058–1061.

Feingold A, Rounsaville B. Construct validity of the dependence syndrome as measured by DSM-IV for different psychoactive substances. Addiction 1995; 90: 1661–1669.

Gossop M, Darke S, Griffiths P, Hando J, Powis B, Hall W, Strang J. The Severity of Dependence Scale (SDS): psychometric properties of the SDS in English and Australian samples of heroin, cocaine and amphetamine users. Addiction 1995; 90: 607–614.

Gossop M, Stewart D, Marsden J. Effectiveness of drug and alcohol counselling during methadone treatment: content, frequency, and duration of counselling and association with substance use outcomes. Addiction 2006; 101: 404–412.

Grant BF, Moore TC, Shepard J, Kaplan K. Source and accuracy statement: Wave I National Epidemiologic Survey on Alcohol and Related Conditions (NESARC). Bethesda, MD: National Institute on Alcohol Abuse and Alcoholism, 2003.

Grant BF, Stinson FS, Dawson DA, Chou SP, Dufour MC, Compton W, Pickering RP, Kaplan K. Prevalence and co-occurrence of substance use disorders and independent mood and anxiety disorders: results from the National Epidemiologic Survey on Alcohol and Related Conditions. Arch Gen Psychiatry 2004; 61: 807–816.

Hall W, Saunders JB, Babor TF, Aasland OG, Amundsen A, Hodgson R, Grant M. The structure and correlates of alcohol dependence: WHO collaborative project on the early detection of persons with harmful alcohol consumption—III. Addiction 1993; 88: 1627–1636.

Harford TC, Muthen BO. The dimensionality of alcohol abuse and dependence: a multivariate analysis of DSM-IV symptom items in the National Longitudinal Survey of Youth. J Stud Alcohol 2001; 62: 150–157.

Hasin DS, Grant BF, Harford TC, Endicott J. The drug dependence syndrome and related disabilities. Br J Addict 1988; 83: 45–55.

Hasin DS, Muthuen B, Wisnicki KS, Grant B. Validity of the bi-axial dependence concept: a test in the U.S. general population. Addiction 1994; 89: 573–579.

Hasin DS, Liu X, Alderson D, Grant BF. DSM-IV alcohol dependence: a categorical or dimensional phenotype? Psychol Med 2006; 36: 1695–1705.

Heath AC, Bucholz KK, Slutske WS, Madden PAF, Dinwiddie SH, Dunne MP, Statham DB, Whitfield JB, Martin NG, Eaves LJ. The assessment of alcoholism in surveys of the general community: what are we measuring? some insights from the Australian twin panel interview survey. Int Rev Psychiatry 1994; 6: 295–307.

Helzer JE, Robins LN, McEvoy LT, Spitznagel EL, Stoltzman RK, Farmer A, Brockington IF. A comparison of clinical and Diagnostic Interview Schedule diagnoses. Physician reexamination of lay-interviewed cases in the general population. Arch Gen Psychiatry 1985; 42: 657–666.

Hughes JR, Oliveto AH, Riggs R, Kenny M, Liguori A, Pillitteri JL, MacLaughlin MA. Concordance of different measures of nicotine dependence: two pilot studies. Addict Behav 2004; 29: 1527–1539.

Jellinek EM. The disease concept of alcoholism. New Brunswick, NY: Hillhouse Press, 1960.

Johnson EO, Breslau N, Anthony JC. The latent dimensionality of DIS/DSM-III-R nicotine dependence: exploratory analyses. Addiction 1996; 91: 583–588.

Kahler CW, Strong DR. A Rasch model analysis of DSM-IV Alcohol abuse and dependence items in the National Epidemiological Survey on Alcohol and Related Conditions. Alcohol Clin Exp Res 2006; 30: 1165–1175.

Kahler CW, Strong DR, Hayaki J, Ramsey SE, Brown RA. An item response analysis of the Alcohol Dependence Scale in treatment-seeking alcoholics. J Stud Alcohol 2003; 64: 127–136.

Kahler CW, Strong DR, Read JP, Palfai TP, Wood MD. Mapping the continuum of alcohol problems in college students: a Rasch model analysis. Psychol Addict Behav 2004; 18: 322–333.

Kalivas PW, Volkow ND. The neural basis of addiction: a pathology of motivation and choice. Am J Psychiatry 2005; 162: 1403–1413.

Kirisci L, Vanyukov M, Dunn M, Tarter R. Item response theory modeling of substance use: an index based on 10 drug categories. Psychol Addict Behav 2002; 16: 290–298.

Kirisci L, Tarter RE, Vanyukov M, Martin C, Mezzich A, Brown S. Application of item response theory to quantify substance use disorder severity. Addict Behav 2006; 31: 1035–1049.

Kosten TR, Rounsaville BJ, Babor TF, Spitzer RL, Williams JB. Substance-use disorders in DSM-III-R. Evidence for the dependence syndrome across different psychoactive substances. Br J Psychiatry 1987; 151: 834–843.

Kraemer HC. DSM categories and dimensions in clinical and research contexts. Int J Methods Psychiatr Res 2007; 16(S1): S8–S15.

Kraemer HC, Noda A, O'Hara R. Categorical versus dimensional approaches to diagnosis: methodological challenges. J Psychiatr Res 2004; 38: 17–25.

Krueger RF, Nichol PE, Hicks BM, Markon KE, Patrick CJ, Iacono WG, McGue M. Using latent trait modeling to conceptualize an alcohol problems continuum. Psychol Assess 2004; 16: 107–119.

Langenbucher JW, Labouvie E, Martin CS, Sanjuan PM, Bavly L, Kirisci L, Chung T. An application of item response theory analysis to alcohol, cannabis, and cocaine criteria in DSM-IV. J Abnorm Psychol 2004; 113: 72–80.

Lanza ST, Flaherty BP, Collins LM. Latent class and latent transition analysis. In JA Schinka, WF Velicer (eds) Handbook of Psychology, Vol 2. Research Methods in Psychology. Hoboken, NJ: John Wiley & Sons, 2003, pp. 663–685.

Lynskey MT, Nelson EC, Neuman RJ, Bucholz KK, Madden PAF, Knopik VS, Slutske W, Whitfield JB, Martin NG, Heath AC. Limitations of DSM-IV operationalizations of alcohol abuse and dependence in a sample of Australian twins. Twin Res Hum Genet 2005; 8: 574–584.

Martin CS, Chung T, Kirisci L, Langenbucher JW. Item response theory analysis of diagnostic criteria for alcohol and cannabis use disorders in adolescents: implications for DSM-V. J Abnorm Psychol 2006; 115: 807–814.

Morey LC, Skinner HA. Empirically derived classifications of alcohol related problems. In Galanter M (ed) Recent developments in alcoholism, Vol IV. New York: Plenum Publishing, 1986, pp. 145–168.

Morey LC, Skinner HA, Blashfield RK. A typology of alcohol abusers: correlates and implications. J Abnorm Psychol 1984; 93: 408–417.

Morgenstern J, Langenbucher J, Labouvie EW. The generalizability of the dependence syndrome across substances: an examination of some properties of the proposed DSM-IV dependence criteria. Addiction 1994; 89: 1105–1113.

Morley KC, Teesson M, Reid SC, Sannibale C, Thomson C, Phung N, Weltman M, Bell JR, Richardson K, Haber PS. Naltrexone versus acamprosate in the treatment of alcohol dependence: a multi-centre, randomized, double-blind, placebo-controlled trial. Addiction 2006; 101: 1451–1462.

Muthen BO. Factor analysis of alcohol abuse and dependence symptom items in the 1988 National Health Interview Survey. Addiction 1995; 90: 637–645.

Muthen BO. Psychometric evaluation of diagnostic criteria: application to a two-dimensional model of alcohol abuse and dependence. Drug Alcohol Depend 1996; 41: 101–112.

Muthen B, Asparouhov T. Item response mixture modeling: application to tobacco dependence criteria. Addict Behav 2006; 31: 1050–1066.

Muthen BO, Grant B, Hasin D. The dimensionality of alcohol abuse and dependence: factor analysis of DSM-III-R and proposed DSM-IV criteria in the 1988 National Health Interview Survey. Addiction 1993a; 88: 1079–1090.

Muthen BO, Hasin D, Wisnicki KS. Factor analysis of ICD-10 symptom items in 1988 National Health Interview Survey on Alcohol Dependence. Addiction 1993b; 88: 1071–1077.

Nelson CB, Rehm J, Ustun TB, Grant B, Chatterji S. Factor structures for DSM-IV substance disorder criteria endorsed by alcohol, cannabis, cocaine and opiate users: results from the WHO reliability and validity study. Addiction 1999; 94: 843–855.

Proudfoot H, Baillie AJ, Teesson M. The structure of alcohol dependence in the community. Drug Alcohol Depend 2006; 81: 21–26.

Radzius A, Gallo J, Gorelick DA, Cadet JL, Uhl G, Henningfield JE, Moolchan ET. Nicotine dependence criteria of the DIS and DSM-III-R: a factor analysis. Nicotine Tob Res 2004; 6: 303–308.

Rohan WP. Quantitative dimensions of alcohol use for hospitalized problem drinkers. Dis Nerv Syst 1976; 37: 154–159.

Saha TD, Chou SP, Grant BF. Toward an alcohol use disorder continuum using item response theory: results from the National Epidemiologic Survey on Alcohol and Related Conditions. Psychol Med 2006; 36: 931–941.

Saha TD, Stinson FS, Grant BF. The role of alcohol consumption in future classifications of alcohol use disorders. Drug Alcohol Depend 2007; 89: 82–92.

Strong DR, Kahler CW, Ramsey SE, Brown RA. Finding order in the DSM-IV nicotine dependence syndrome: a Rasch analysis. Drug Alcohol Depend 2003; 72: 151–162.

Teesson M, Lynskey M, Manor B, Baillie A. The structure of cannabis dependence in the community. Drug Alcohol Depend 2002; 68: 255–262.

World Health Organization (WHO). Severity of Dependence Scale (SDS). Available online: http://www.who.int/substance_ abuse/research_tools/severitydependencescale/ en (12 December 2006). Adapted from: Gossop M, Darke S, Griffiths P, Hando J, Powis B, Hall W, Strang J. The Severity of Dependence Scale (SDS): psychometric properties of the SDS in English and Australian samples of heroin, cocaine and amphetamine users. Addiction 1995; 90: 607–614.

# 4

# DIMENSIONALITY AND THE CATEGORY OF MAJOR DEPRESSIVE EPISODE

Gavin Andrews, M.D.
Traolach Brugha, M.D.
Michael E. Thase, M.D.
Farifteh Firoozmand Duffy, Ph.D.
Paola Rucci, Ph.D.
Timothy Slade, Ph.D.

Major depressive episode (MDE) is a common syndrome comprising depression, loss of interest, and other symptoms. There are no laboratory tests for MDE, and diagnosis depends on a trained clinician asking people about their symptoms. The American Psychiatric Association's *Diagnostic and Statistical Manual of Mental Disorders,* Fourth Edition (DSM-IV; American Psychiatric Association 1994) criteria consist of nine symptoms, five of which must be present and at least one of the five must be "depressed mood" or "loss of interest or pleasure" for the diagnosis to be met. All must be judged by an experienced clinician to be significant in terms of severity, duration, abnormality, distress, and impairment. These symptoms, we will argue, exist on a continuum, and the 5/9 DSM symptoms are an arbitrary point above which diagnosis is made and medical intervention is deemed appropriate (Table 4–1).

Reprinted with permission from Andrews G, Brugha T, Thase ME, Duffy FF, Rucci P, Slade T. "Dimensionality and the Category of Major Depressive Episode." *International Journal of Methods in Psychiatric Research* 2007; 16(S1): S41–S51.

# The Epidemiology of Depression

Depressive symptoms in the population are common, but having symptoms is not the same thing as meeting criteria for a depressive disorder. In the Australian survey, 17% of adults reported at least 2 weeks of depressed mood or loss of interest in the past year, but only 6.3% met the full DSM-IV criteria at some point in the year prior to the survey, and only 3.2% were current cases.

Depression occurs throughout the life span and is more common in women. What proportion of the population will have an episode of depression? In the U.S. National Comorbidity Survey, 17% had met criteria but the average age was only 34 so only half of the age of risk had passed (Kessler et al. 1996). A modeling study, using Australian and Dutch data and allowing for age of respondent and recall bias, estimated the lifetime risk of at least one episode of major depression as 30% for males and 40% for females (Kruijshaar et al. 2005). On the basis of prospective studies, others have estimated the lifetime risk to be higher (Andrews et al. 2005).

Depression is a disorder that remits and recurs. At the severe end of the spectrum, two 15-year prospective studies of people admitted to the hospital with depression found these patients did not fare well (Kiloh et al. 1988; Lee and Murray 1988). Only a fifth of these people hospitalized for depression recovered and remained continuously well; three-fifths recovered but also had further episodes; a tenth were lost to suicide; and a tenth were always incapacitated. A 12-year study in U.S. specialist care, again presumably of people with severe illness, showed that patients had symptoms in 60% of follow-up weeks and met full criteria for a depressive episode in 15% of those weeks (Judd et al. 1998). This is one of the few studies that have documented the level of subthreshold and threshold depression in a cohort followed for a substantial period. Cuijpers and Smit (2004) have assembled a series of studies that show that people with subthreshold symptoms have, compared to people without symptoms, a fivefold increase in risk of developing MDE.

Depression is usually episodic. The U.S. National Comorbidity Survey showed that three-quarters of people aged 15–54 years who had ever met criteria for depression had had more than one episode. Their mean age was 34, and they reported an average of four episodes in the 11 years since their first episode (Kessler et al. 1996). The World Health Organization (WHO) Global Burden of Disease 2000 study estimated a mean episode duration of 26 weeks (Ustun et al. 2004), and the literature is consistent with this. The median duration of an episode is less, around 13 weeks.

To summarize: If depressive episodes have a mean duration of about 6 months, some episodes will last weeks, others (perhaps 5%–10%) will not remit for some years. As some will suicide, we will never know when they would have remitted. Episodes recur, with the average number of episodes predicted from community survey data being around eight in a person's lifetime. Thus the average person with depression can expect to meet criteria for a depressive episode for some 4 years in a lifetime. In addition, judging from the data on more severe cases, patients will report symp-

---

**TABLE 4–1.** Summary of DSM-IV criteria for major depressive episode

---

Five or more symptoms present during the same 2-week period, including
either 1 or 2:

1. Depressed mood

2. Loss of interest or pleasure

3. Significant weight loss or gain

4. Insomnia or hypersomnia

5. Psychomotor agitation or retardation

6. Fatigue or loss of energy

7. Feelings of worthlessness or excessive or inappropriate guilt

8. Diminished ability to think, concentrate, or make decisions

9. Recurrent thoughts of death, recurrent suicidal ideation, or suicide attempt
   or plan

The symptoms must persist for most of the day, nearly every day within the
2-week period, be a change from the person's usual state, and must involve
clinically significant distress or impairment in functioning (e.g., occupational
or social).

---

toms of depression that do not meet criteria for a diagnosis but nevertheless are associated with some disability for three or four times as long, that is, for 12–16 years
in a lifetime. But provided they do not commit suicide, they can expect 60 years in
a lifetime without depressive symptoms, including some 35 years of working life.
Nevertheless, depressive illness is common and can be very disabling.

# The Diagnosis of Depression

A disease is a harmful state that is, or could be, of clinical relevance. The purpose
of medicine is to reduce the burden of human disease by reducing risk factors, by
educating people how to manage themselves, and by the direct treatment of disease in patients who seek help. Mental diseases are called disorders, if only because
we remain unsure of the disease processes that underlie the disorders. To quote
Kraemer (Chapter 2), a diagnosis of a disorder is a "clinical expert's opinion" that
the disorder is present. Clearly the disorder was present before the expert clinician
made the diagnosis, and it will still be present when treatment has reduced the
symptoms on which the diagnosis was based. When the disorder began, it was
probably mild and would not have satisfied the formal diagnostic criteria; after effective treatment, it probably does not satisfy the criteria any longer, but it would
be specious to argue that the disorder changed simply because it failed to match
the threshold required for the formal diagnosis. The purpose of a diagnostic sys-

tem like DSM-IV is simply to describe common patient presentations of a disorder in ways that might help a clinician to recognize the disorder, educate the patient, and apply an effective treatment to produce a better outcome.

The symptoms of MDE listed in Table 4–1 all exist on dimensions of greater or lesser intensity, persistence over time, change in usual state, distress, and impairment. It is the clinician's task to judge whether the severity, duration, abnormality, distress, and impairment of the elicited symptoms warrant the assignment to a diagnostic category, that is, the symptoms exceed a hypothetical threshold in this multidimensional space whereby a diagnosis can be justified and lead to a course of beneficial action. If all this seems complex, it is. Clinical training is about developing the expertise to differentiate significant symptoms from everyday expressions; for example: "It would be better if I was dead" is a serious communication, whereas "I could honestly die" ("Adelaide's Lament" in *Guys and Dolls*) is a nonpathological expression of chagrin. The surprise is firstly that this complex task can be done reliably by well-trained clinicians, and secondly that we have been able to develop structured diagnostic interviews and questionnaires like the Patient Health Questionnaire (PHQ-9) that reliably emulate this process (see Figure 4–3 later in this chapter in the section on the PHQ-9).

The first *International Classification of Diseases* (ICD) was written at the beginning of the last century, when countries needed a standard way of naming the causes of death. The tenth revision of this classification was organized by WHO (World Health Organization 1993). ICD-10 and DSM-IV were designed in parallel and describe the diagnostic criteria for the same range of mental disorders. While there are differences of detail, the similarities were so great that an international edition of DSM-IV was published that was able to apply the ICD-10 diagnostic codes to the DSM-IV diagnostic criteria. Remember that no one can show a mental disorder like a surgeon can show an excised tumor, and so the classifications describe phenomenology, the different changes in thoughts, emotions, and behaviors thought to be characteristic of each mental disorder. Neither classification included changes at the cellular level for any criteria. To reiterate, experts from all over the world were able to agree on the taxonomy of mental disorders that afflicted the human race and on the criteria that health services could use to diagnose people with these distinct disorders. Depression, therefore, was regarded as a category of disorder for which treatment could be indicated. Five of nine on a dimension of nine symptoms was the threshold above which MDE could be diagnosed.

# Evidence for the Dimensionality of Depression

## THE DISTRIBUTION OF SYMPTOMS

The idea of a threshold on a continuum of symptoms is not new. At the lower end of the intelligence distributions in general populations there is a clear excess of cases that represent the distinct pathology of severe mental retardation. Therefore, a recent study aimed to establish whether such subpopulations exist in distributions of common mental disorders (mixed anxiety and depression current symptoms), above epidemiological "case" cutoffs. Data from 9,556 non-psychotic respondents to the 1993 Office of Population Censuses and Surveys National Household Psychiatric Morbidity Survey were analyzed (Melzer et al. 2002). The program of surveys includes general population surveys of adults living in the community in Great Britain. The principal United Kingdom survey diagnostic interview used the revised Clinical Interview Schedule (Lewis et al. 1992) to collect data about common psychiatric symptoms. This schedule yielded standardized quantitative (i.e., dimensional) scores and diagnostic categories, for which additional information needed for diagnostic criteria was also collected.

The symptom scores, when combined into a single score, yield an operational definition of a case—a cutoff of 12 or more symptoms being conventionally used for this purpose. The distribution of total neurotic symptom and depression scores from the revised Clinical Interview Schedule was examined. Automated least squares methods were used to fit the best single statistical distribution to the data (Figure 4–1). A single exponential curve provided the best fit for the whole population, but floor effects produced deviations at symptom counts of 0–3 (two in three respondents in the general population had no current symptoms). After truncation, exponential distributions fitted the symptom data excellently. Proportions of the population above the conventional cutoffs of 12 or more symptoms differed by less than 12% from expected for a range of low- and high-prevalence groups. These low- and high-prevalence groups were also then identified by the presence or absence of putative risk factors such as recent stressful life events. Symptom counts for the common mental disorders fall within single population distributions, with little apparent numerical excess in the case range. High and low prevalences of these disorders appear to be population characteristics, with shifts in exponential means predicting proportions above case cutoffs. The single exponential model also fitted the depression scores alone.

## IS THERE A DISCONTINUITY AT 5/9 SYMPTOMS?

This prompts an important question: is there any evidence of a natural break in the distribution of symptoms at or around the threshold between four or fewer and five or more symptoms? This issue has been explored in a number of ways. Kessler et al. (1997), using data from the National Comorbidity Survey, examined the relationship between groups, defined by the number of depressive symptoms and risk of multiple clinical correlates, including parental history of mental illness, number or duration of depressive episodes, and comorbidity. They found that the risk of these clinical correlates increased with increasing numbers of symptoms. Ustun and Sartorius (1995) led a study of 5,000 primary care attend-

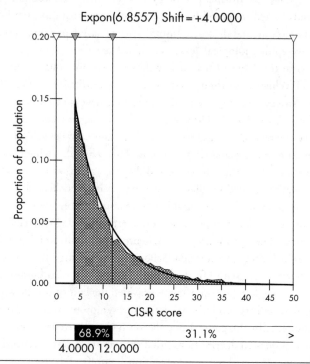

**FIGURE 4–1.** Proportion of population by full range of CIS-R scores, and fitted exponential curve. Goodness of fit (RMS error) test statistic=0.0286E-04.

*Note.* CIS-R=Revised Clinical Interview Schedule; RMS=root mean square.

*Source.* Reprinted from Melzer D, Tom BD, Brugha TS, et al. "Common Mental Disorder Symptom Counts in Populations: Are There Distinct Case Groups Above Epidemiological Cut-Offs?" *Psychological Medicine* 2002; 32: 1195–1201, with permission of Cambridge University Press. Copyright © 2002, Cambridge University Press.

ees in 14 countries and found a linear relation between disability and number of depression symptoms. Sakashita et al. (2007) selected all people who endorsed the symptoms of either "sadness or loss of interest" in the Australian National Survey of Mental Health and Well-Being (NSMHWB) and examined the distribution of the remaining seven possible symptoms of depression as predictors of four measures of impairment. The relationship between the number of symptoms and impairment was linear, with no evidence of any natural discontinuity that would support the use of 5/9 symptoms as a diagnostic threshold.

Both these studies examine the manifest or observable relationship between the number of depressive symptoms and suggested validators of disease. However, recent focus has shifted to investigation of the latent structure of constructs such as depression. These studies concentrate on the internal relationship between symptoms of depression and how these relationships give rise to the surface expression of symptomatology. Slade and Andrews (2005) examined the latent structure of depression in the Australian NSMHWB using taxometric analysis, a statistical technique designed specifically to determine whether a given construct is best conceptualized by two latent discrete categories or one latent continuous dimension. They concluded, as had Ruscio and Ruscio (2000) before them, that depression is best conceptualized, measured, and classified as a continuously distributed syndrome rather than as a discrete diagnostic entity. One of the implications of this finding is that the decision to offer treatment can be made at any level on the continuum.

## CORRELATES OF SEVERITY

Although major depressive disorder is a categorical classification (i.e., patients either meet criteria for the diagnosis or they do not), a number of relevant dimensions convey useful information about the individual's clinical state. Among these, a unitary dimension of symptom severity is arguably the most important, conveying valuable descriptive and prognostic information. Clinical correlates of high pretreatment severity include suicidality, melancholic and psychotic features, and various types of comorbidity (i.e., anxiety disorders, high scores on trait-like measures of neuroticism and dysfunctional attitudes, and increased likelihood of selected Cluster B and C personality disorders). Likewise, as depression symptom severity increases, the probability of biological correlates of dysphoric activation increases. Neurobiological correlates include hypercortisolism, changes in regional cerebral metabolism (increased activation of amygdala, decreased activation of prefrontal cortical structures), and increased peripheral levels of norepinephrine metabolites. Increased symptom severity has important treatment implications, such as a lower likelihood of responding to an acute phase therapy, longer time to remission and recovery, a relatively lower likelihood of placebo response compared to antidepressant response, and a greater likelihood of response to combined psychotherapy and pharmacotherapy compared to therapy with either alone. These differences can be large and very clinically meaningful. For example, in a meta-analysis of individual patient data pooled from six different studies conducted at the University of Pittsburgh Medical Center in the 1980s, Thase et al. (1997) found that whereas the combination of antidepressant medication and psychotherapy had a modest advantage over psychotherapy alone for patients with milder depressive episodes (i.e., about a 10% difference in remission rates), among those with moderate to severe levels of pretreatment severity, the advantage of receiving both medication and psychotherapy was a nearly 30% advantage in remission rates as compared to treatment with psychotherapy alone.

It is becoming clear that mental disorders are best described in terms of dimensions; doctors do have to make binary decisions—i.e., to treat or not. But the idea that psychiatrists should only use categorical diagnoses may also be based on the misconceived idea that this is what physicians actually do. Best current practice for the medical management of cardiovascular risk prediction recommends the use of a range of dimensional or continuous assessments of blood pressure and cholesterol high-density lipoprotein ratio, a recommendation that is widely disseminated to United Kingdom medical practitioners through the regularly updated British National Formulary (2000). Levels of severity of depression below and above the conventional diagnostic threshold are also being used nationally for treatment decisions based on explicit ICD-10 criteria for depressive episode and disorder, which is closely equivalent to major depression. The National Centre for Clinical Excellence in the United Kingdom recommends that while the decision to treat could be made in all cases of depression, the response would be stepped or graded according to severity of the depression as operationally defined in ICD-10. That is, while mild cases would be offered "watchful waiting and guided self-help," moderate cases would be offered medication and psychological therapies and very severe cases, in which there was a risk to life, would be offered inpatient care and treatments, including medication, psychological therapies, and/or electroconvulsive therapy (ECT). People with symptoms of depression that do not meet the diagnostic threshold are regarded as not needing treatment at all, as though there was a categorical difference between them and those with mild depression.

## THE LATENT STRUCTURE OF MENTAL DISORDERS

If the boundaries of MDE shade into "normal" depression, are the boundaries between it and related mental disorders distinct? If this were indeed the case, then the rates of co-occurrence among individual mental disorders would occur at, or around, chance levels. However, the rates of co-occurrence among the mental disorders are higher than would be expected by chance (Andrews 1996; Andrews et al. 2002). It has been suggested that such rates could reflect the existence of higher order dimensions of psychopathology. A number of studies have examined this and found consistent and meaningful groupings of mental disorders (Kessler et al. 2005; Krueger 1999). Using methodology originally outlined in Krueger (1999), the most recent of these studies (Slade and Watson 2006) identified a hierarchical three-factor structure as the best fit to 10 common DSM-IV and 11 common ICD-10 mental disorders. This structure was characterized by a distress and a fear factor (which were best considered lower order facets of a broader internalizing factor), as well as an externalizing factor. As can be seen in Figure 4–2, the individual mental disorders that were characteristic of the distress factor were major depression, dysthymia, generalized anxiety disorder, posttraumatic stress disorder and neurasthenia (in the ICD-10 model). The mental disorders that were characteristic of the fear factor were social phobia, agoraphobia, panic disorder, and obsessive-compulsive disorder. The externalizing factor was best characterized by drug and alcohol dependence.

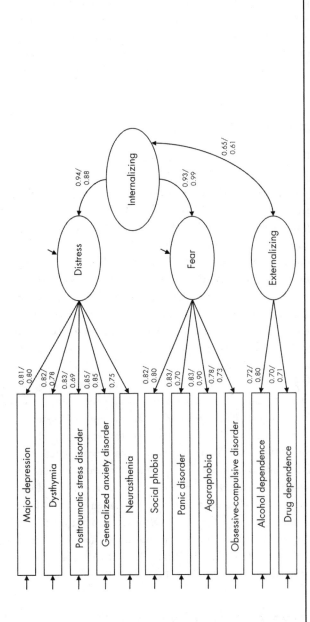

**FIGURE 4–2.**     Best-fitting model of the structure of 10 common DSM-IV and 11 common ICD-10 mental disorders from the Australian National Survey of Mental Health and Well-Being (NSMHWB), 1997.

All parameter estimates (DSM-IV/ICD-10) are standardized and significant at *P*<0.05. All parameter estimates, except for neurasthenia, relate to DSM-IV/ICD-10. The single parameter estimate for neurasthenia relates to ICD-10 only.

*Source.*   Reprinted from Slade T, Watson D. "The Structure of Common DSM-IV and ICD-10 Mental Disorders in the Australian General Population." *Psychological Medicine* 2006; 36: 1593–1600, with permission of Cambridge University Press. Copyright © 2006, Cambridge University Press.

It has been supposed that as genetic and brain structure and functioning information became more precise, it would support the existence of categories of mental disorders. This has not yet proved to be the case. The genetic underpinnings of depression are probably more related to the higher order dimensions of psychopathology demonstrated earlier than to the individual syndromes. The information from brain function and structure appears to be similar.

## ONE DIMENSION OR MANY?

The diagnosis of MDE depends on a clinician identifying the number and severity of symptoms, their duration, abnormality, and the resulting distress and impairment. Most patients seek help because their symptoms have resulted in impairment and most clinicians make a diagnosis on the basis of the abnormal nature of the 5–9 symptoms that the patient describes. Are all these elements present in all cases? In data from the Australian National Survey (Andrews et al. 2001) there were cases who met criteria for current MDE who reported being satisfied with life, or who were not distressed or disabled. In fact, about 20% of people who were currently depressed reported that they were delighted, pleased, or mostly satisfied with life. Compared to the remainder of cases, this minority was more likely to have only five symptoms, have a lower neuroticism score, and report fewer comorbid conditions and lower levels of help-seeking characteristics, similar to those with subthreshold conditions (Table 4–2).

This is further evidence of the dimensional nature of MDE within a higher order of distress disorders. If remission in particular and prognosis in general depends on symptom severity, then clinicians need an instrument to allow them to easily document the level of severity and the response to treatment. While the number of depressive symptoms is highly correlated with the measures of well-being, distress, disability, and neuroticism mentioned earlier (and the four measures listed do inform about aspects of patient status that are not captured by the diagnosis alone), there are a number of people who meet criteria for mild MDE who express themselves as pleased with life, or not distressed, or not disabled, or not normally nervous. Clearly these measures are inappropriate as clinical indicators of the main dimensional nature of MDE. The Patient Health Questionnaire is derived from the diagnostic criteria and does not suffer from this limitation.

# The Patient Health Questionnaire–9

The nine-item Patient Health Questionnaire (PHQ-9; see Figure 4–3) is a patient self-report instrument that parallels the symptom criteria for depressive disorders listed in DSM-IV. It is one option that could introduce some dimensionality into DSM-V without a radical alteration in the diagnostic criteria. The dimensionality is

**TABLE 4–2.** Responses of the 10,641 respondents to the Australian National Survey of Mental Health and Well-Being (NSMHWB) on a scale of well-being[a] against the probability of having a current ICD-10 diagnosis of major depression and of being significantly disabled (SF-12), distressed (K10), or having a high neuroticism score (EPQ short form)

| Delighted terrible scale[a] | ICD-10 major depression Last 1-month, N=423 weighted % (SD) | SF-12 Mental scale score is greater than 1 SD below mean weighted % (SD) | K-10 (psychological distress score)>20 (indicating likely to have mild, moderate, or severe mental disorder) weighted % (SD) | EPQ-Neuroticism scale score > 1 SD from the mean score observed for NSMHWB respondents weighted % (SD) |
|---|---|---|---|---|
| 1 (Delighted) N=1,102 | 0.8 (0.3) positive n=10 | 11.1 (1.1) positive n=129 | 2.7 (0.5) positive n=32 | 6.9 (0.9) positive n=79 |
| 2 (Pleased) N=3,140 | 0.6 (0.1) positive n=25 | 15.9 (0.8) positive n=502 | 4.4 (0.4) positive n=140 | 11.1 (0.5) positive n=351 |
| 3 (Mostly satisfied) N=3,893 | 1.4 (0.2) positive n=60 | 24.7 (0.7) positive n=952 | 7.6 (0.6) positive n=284 | 18.1 (0.7) positive n=686 |
| 4 (Mixed) N=1,943 | 7.5 (0.6) positive n=166 | 55.1 (1.0) positive n=1,077 | 27.7 (0.9) positive n=532 | 40.5 (1.4) positive n=795 |
| 5 (Mostly dissatisfied) N=305 | 16.3 (2.5) positive n=54 | 79.8 (2.8) positive n=243 | 55.0 (3.4) positive n=167 | 59.6 (4.0) positive n=179 |
| 6 (Unhappy) N=180 | 37.0 (3.9) positive n=77 | 83.7 (3.4) positive n=153 | 62.3 (4.1) positive n=126 | 67.2 (4.1) positive n=125 |
| 7 (Terrible) N=78 | 42.0 (6.7) positive n=31 | 90.4 (4.6) positive n=70 | 75.3 (4.4) positive n=59 | 75.9 (4.3) positive n=60 |

[a]Andrews and Withey 1976.
*Note.* SD =standard deviation.

## PATIENT HEALTH QUESTIONNAIRE (PHQ-9)

### English

This questionnaire is an important part of providing you with the best health care possible. Your answers will help in understanding problems that you may have. Please answer every question to the best of your ability unless you are requested to skip a question.

Name:_____Age:_____

Sex:  ❑ Female  ❑ Male   Today's Date:_____  _____

Over the <u>last 2 weeks</u> , how often have you been bothered by any of the following problems?

| | Not at all | Several days | More than half the days | Nearly every day |
|---|---|---|---|---|
| | 0 | 1 | 2 | 3 |
| 1. Little interest or pleasure in doing things | ❑ | ❑ | ❑ | ❑ |
| 2. Feeling down, depressed, or hopeless | ❑ | ❑ | ❑ | ❑ |
| 3. Trouble falling or staying asleep, or sleeping too much | ❑ | ❑ | ❑ | ❑ |
| 4. Feeling tired or having little energy | ❑ | ❑ | ❑ | ❑ |
| 5. Poor appetite or overeating | ❑ | ❑ | ❑ | ❑ |
| 6. Feeling bad about yourself, or that you are a failure, or have let yourself or your family down | ❑ | ❑ | ❑ | ❑ |
| 7. Trouble concentrating on things, such as reading the newspaper or watching television | ❑ | ❑ | ❑ | ❑ |
| 8. Moving or speaking so slowly that other people could have noticed. Or the opposite—being so fidgety or restless that you have been moving around a lot more than usual | ❑ | ❑ | ❑ | ❑ |
| 9. Thoughts that you would be better off dead, or of hurting yourself in some way | ❑ | ❑ | ❑ | ❑ |

If you checked "several days" or higher for some of the questions above, discuss your answers with a doctor Only a doctor can make a diagnosis of depression. Also talk to your doctor if you checked "several days" or higher for (9), thinking that you would be better off dead or wanting to hurt yourself. Having repeated thoughts of death or suicide is the most serious symptom of depression. If you are thinking of harming yourself, get helpimmediately, make your feelings known to someone who can help you—your doctor, family members, friends. Your doctor is an excellent person to tell.

KEY (for physician's use): MDD if answer to # 1 or 2 and 5 or more of # 1-9 are at least "More than half the days" (count # 9 if present at all).

**FIGURE 4–3.**   The Patient Health Questionnaire (PHQ-9).

*Source.*   Copyright © 2005 Pfizer, Inc. All rights reserved. Used with permission. Can be downloaded from http://www.phqscreeners.com/pdfs/PHQ-9/English.pdf.

achieved because each symptom is extended to include four levels of severity based on the frequency of the symptoms over a 2-week period. The respondent is asked, "Over the last two weeks, how often have you been bothered by any of the following problems?" and is given four choice options for each nine symptoms: 0 = not at all; 1 = for several days; 2 = more than half the days; 3 = nearly every day. The total score, which must be validated by a clinician, can therefore range between 0 and 27. Depression severity is judged from the total score as follows: 0–4 None, 5–9 Mild, 10–14 Moderate, 15–19 Moderately severe, 20–27 Severe (http://www.pfizer.com/phq-9; Kroenke and Spitzer 2002). Because of its brevity and sensitivity to change over time, the PHQ-9 can be used for screening new patients for depression as well as for routine use in evaluating outcome and response to treatment. There are longer and more detailed scales available, but the PHQ-9 is recommended as being simple, acceptable to patients, and practical for clinicians to use. It is, within the bounds set by self-report, brief, reliable, and valid (Kroenke et al. 2001).

Based on the PHQ-9 diagnostic instructions, a diagnosis of major depressive disorder can be achieved when at least one of the first two questions (feeling depressed, little pleasure) is endorsed for more than half the days or nearly every day in the past 2 weeks together with four other symptoms endorsed at a similar range for intensity. Other depressive disorders may be considered if there are two to four symptom criteria endorsed for more than half the days or nearly every day, one of which corresponds to depressed feeling or loss of interest or pleasure. Item 9, which concerns suicidal thoughts, counts as a positive if present at all, regardless of its duration (Kroenke and Spitzer 2002).

In employing the PHQ-9 to introduce dimensionality into depression diagnoses, it is important to make note of potential sources for misclassification. For example, if neither of the questions on depressed feelings or loss of interest is endorsed, but the scores on other symptom criteria add up to 10 or more, a diagnosis of depression cannot be achieved. Similarly, if one symptom is endorsed at "more than half the days" level and all other eight symptoms are endorsed at the "several days" level (totaling to 10), an individual may not technically qualify for moderate severity of depression according to the PHQ-9 instructions, although presence of suicidal thoughts certainly needs to be further probed. Therefore, in marginal cases, review by trained clinical staff is essential.

When used to assess treatment response, a drop of five points from baseline after 4–6 weeks of treatment qualifies as a clinically significant response, whereas a drop of less than two points is considered inadequate and indicates the need for a review of treatment. An absolute PHQ-9 score of less than 10 is considered a partial response, and a score of less than five qualifies as remission (Kroenke and Spitzer 2002). Patients may complete the scale at home and telephone the results to the clinic or bring in the completed form during each scheduled appointment.

The PHQ-9 does have limitations. It does not cover the symptoms associated with the complex forms of depression nor with comorbid or mixed states. It is not yet validated in youth, nor is it available in very many languages. Its brevity and its dual use in making a diagnosis and assessing severity and improvement of depressive disorders are great advantages, but at a cost in terms of its sensitivity and comprehensiveness. Nevertheless, a combined assessment of depression diagnosis and severity can support clinicians in screening and identify probable cases, in focusing clinical attention or providing timely referral for severely depressed patients, and in providing care to less severely impaired patients who need treatment (Nease and Malouin 2003).

In a study by Spitzer et al. (1999), 87% of primary care physicians rated the diagnostic information provided by the PHQ-9 as somewhat or very useful in management and treatment planning. The investigators found that 22% of patients with a PHQ-9 diagnosis of major depression had follow-up visits, 10% were prescribed antidepressants, and 5% were referred to mental health professionals (Spitzer et al. 1999). In a recent study, psychiatrists rated PHQ-9 score as helpful in their treatment decisions in 93% of contacts for patients with depressive disorders. In those instances, the overall PHQ-9 score or item review led to a treatment change for 40% of contacts (e.g., change in dose of antidepressant, adding other medications, starting or increasing psychotherapy, switching antidepressants, etc.), while in 60% of encounters with patients, the score affirmed the benefits of continuing a course of treatment (Katzelnick et al. 2003).

## IMPLICATIONS OF A DIMENSIONAL APPROACH

If the PHQ-9 was approved as part of DSM-V, then there could be a number of consequences. Firstly, we contend that the recognition and treatment of people with depression would improve. Secondly, people would become alert to their depression levels and be able to actively participate in treatment. Thirdly, the seriousness with which the media and the general public view the concept of "major depressive disorder" (MDD) could be challenged. Depression is a normal affect and it is conceivable that many members of the general public who have been depressed believe they know all there is to know about depressive disorders. Some symptoms of depression are tolerable, and the general pubic would like to believe that mental illness is not a great issue. The publication of a self-administered test could compound this situation, because they will be able to complete the PHQ-9 and match symptoms that have been present to a mild degree with the symptoms required to meet criteria for MDD, and falsely claim that they know that depression is not usually that terrible. We therefore contend that the ancillary information offered in DSM-V should contain information about the epidemiology of MDE listed at the beginning of this chapter.

There are other implications that stem from a dimensional (and open) approach to diagnosis. Clinicians use categories to facilitate brief and efficient communication with colleagues and to organize treatment. They also use a dimensional approach for the same purpose, whether they are presenting a full formulation that identifies a patient's strengths and weaknesses, just identifying the severity, or noting the change in severity with treatment. The PHQ-9 will facilitate each of these steps. The idea that most disorders are dimensional may raise political questions. For example, funders currently use categories, but dimensions would be more applicable if payment was titrated to the degree of difficulty likely in treatment. Many diagnosis-related group classifications already have a primitive dimensional aspect related to treatment difficulty. Similarly, lawyers already use dimensions. Journalists will prefer categories for a brief news item but will understand the value of the dimensional approach for a longer opinion piece.

The introduction of measures like the PHQ-9 is a modest step towards dimensionality and will have several very positive advantages. Firstly, as was shown in the section on the PHQ-9, it facilitates treatment, both confirming the continuation of an effective treatment and stimulating the change to an alternative treatment when the first choice is not working. Other advantages are more theoretical. Dimensional data provide links to higher order dimensions that may be of considerable importance to the understanding of the pathogenesis, course, and co-occurrence of emotional disorders (Brown et al. 1998). Dimensional data may also contribute to the precision of the diagnosis of depression and identify subtypes of individuals who require different treatment strategies. Using a broader dimensional assessment of mood spectrum that includes DSM-IV criteria for mood disorders and associated features, Cassano et al. (2004) found that in depressed patients without a history of hypomania according to the DSM-IV criteria, the occurrence of manic-hypomanic spectrum symptoms was associated with increased levels of suicidality and paranoid/delusional thoughts.

There is consensus that the distress disorders are associated with negative emotionality. The four disorders in the anxious-misery set, i.e., MDE, dysthymia, bipolar disorder, and generalized anxiety disorder, can be amenable to a dimensional approach. The PHQ-9, we suggest, will describe the dimension of MDE, dysthymia, and the depressed phase of bipolar disorder; the Penn State Worry Questionnaire will describe generalized anxiety disorder; and the Altman Self-Rating Mania Scale (Altman et al. 1997) will describe the acute phase of bipolar disorder. There are self-report measures that would provide comparable information about the fear disorders and the substance use disorders, both generally and specifically, but they are beyond the scope of this chapter.

## Conclusions

MDE refers to an agreed threshold on a dimension of a set number of symptoms. It is argued that the use of a matching scale like the PHQ-9 that establishes the presence and frequency of each individual symptom would facilitate recognition, guide treatment, and be acceptable to consumers, providers, and funders.

# References

Altman E, Hedeker D, Peterson JL, Davis JM. The Altman Self-Rating Mania Scale. Biol Psychiatry 1997; 42: 948–955.

American Psychiatric Association. Diagnostic and Statistical Manual of Mental Disorders, 4th Edition. Washington, DC: American Psychiatric Association, 1994.

Andrews FM, Withey SB. Social Indicators of Well-Being. New York: Plenum Press, 1976.

Andrews G. Comorbidity and the general neurotic syndrome. Br J Psychiatry Suppl 1996; 168: 76–84.

Andrews G, Henderson S, Hall W. Prevalence, comorbidity, disability and service utilisation. Overview of the Australian National Mental Health Survey. Br J Psychiatry 2001; 178: 145–153.

Andrews G, Slade T, Issakidis C. Deconstructing current comorbidity: data from the Australian National Survey of Mental Health and Well-Being. Br J Psychiatry 2002; 181: 306–314.

Andrews G, Poulton R, Skoog I. Lifetime risk of depression: restricted to a minority or waiting for most? Br J Psychiatry 2005; 187: 495–496.

British National Formulary, 40th Edition. London: British Medical Association and the Royal Pharmaceutical Society of Great Britain, 2000.

Brown TA, Chorpita BF, Barlow DH. Structural relationships among dimensions of the DSM-IV anxiety and mood disorders and dimensions of negative affect, positive affect, and autonomic arousal. J Abnorm Psychol 1998; 107: 179–192.

Cassano GB, Rucci P, Frank E, Fagiolini A, Dell'Osso L, Shear MK, Kupfer DJ. The mood spectrum in unipolar and bipolar disorder: arguments for a unitary approach. Am J Psychiatry 2004; 161(7): 1264–1269.

Cuijpers P, Smit F. Subthreshold depression as a risk indicator for major depressive disorder: a systematic review of prospective studies. Acta Psychiatr Scand 2004; 109: 325–331.

Judd LL, Hagop SA, Maser JD, Zeller PJ, et al. A prospective 12 year study of subsyndromal and syndromal depressive symptoms in unipolar major depressive disorders. Arch Gen Psychiatry 1998; 55: 604–700.

Katzelnick D, Chung H, Trivedi M, Duffy FF, Rae D, Regier DA. Use of quantitative instruments for monitoring depression severity: clinical applications. Presentation at the National Depression Management Leadership Initiative: Improving Depression Care Symposium, 156th annual meeting of the American Psychiatric Association, San Francisco, May 17–22, 2003.

Kessler RC, Nelson CB, McGonagle KA, Edlund MJ, Frank RG, Leaf PJ. The epidemiology of co-occurring addictive and mental disorders: implications for prevention and service utilization. Am J Orthopsychiatry 1996; 66: 17–31.

Kessler RC, Zhao S, Blazer DG, Swartz M. Prevalence, correlates, and course of minor depression and major depression in the National Comorbidity Survey. J Affect Disord 1997; 45: 19–30.

Kessler RC, Chiu WT, Demler JJ, Walters EE. Prevalence, severity, and comorbidity of 12-month DSM-IV disorders in the National Comorbidity Survey Replication. Arch Gen Psychiatry 2005; 62: 617–627.

Kiloh LG, Andrews G, Neilson M. The long-term outcome of depressive illness. Br J Psychiatry 1988; 153: 752–757.

Kroenke K, Spitzer RL. The PHQ-9: a new depression diagnostic and severity measure. Psychiatr Ann 2002; 32: 1–7.

Kroenke K, Spitzer RL, Williams JBW. The PHQ-9: validity of a brief depression severity measure. J Gen Intern Med 2001; 16: 606–613.

Krueger RF. The structure of common mental disorders. Arch Gen Psychiatry 1999; 56: 921–926.

Kruijshaar ME, Barendregt J, Vos T, de Graaf R, Spijker J, Andrews G. Lifetime prevalence estimates of major depression: an indirect estimation method and a quantification of recall bias. Eur J Epidemiol 2005; 20: 103–111.

Lee AS, Murray RM. The long term outcome of Maudsley depressives. Br J Psychiatry 1988; 153: 741– 751.

Lewis G, Pelosi AJ, Araya R, Duna G. Measuring psychiatric disorder in the community: a standardized assessment for use by lay interviewers. Psychol Med 1992; 22: 465–486.

Melzer D, Tom BD, Brugha TS, Fryers TF, Meltzer H. Common mental disorder symptom counts in populations: are there distinct case groups above epidemiological cut-offs? Psychol Med 2002; 32(7): 1195–1201.

Nease DE, Malouin JM. Depression screening: a practical strategy. J Family Practice 2003; 52: 118–24.

Patient Health Questionnaire (PHQ-9). Available at: http://www.phqscreeners.com/pdfs/PHQ-9/English.pdf. Accessed January 29, 2008.

Ruscio J, Ruscio AM. Informing the continuity controversy: a taxometric analysis of depression. J Abnorm Psychol 2000; 109: 473–487.

Sakashita C, Slade T, Andrews G. Empirical investigation of two assumptions in the diagnosis of DSM-IV major depressive episode. Aust N Z J Psychiatry 2007; 41: 17–23.

Slade T, Andrews G. Latent structure of depression in a community sample: a taxometric analysis. Psychol Med 2005; 35: 489–497.

Slade T, Watson D. The structure of common DSM-IV and ICD-10 mental disorders in the Australian general population. Psychol Med 2006; 36: 1593–1600.

Spitzer RL, Kroenke K, Williams JBW. Validation and utility of a self-report version of PRIME-MD: the PHQ primary care study. JAMA 1999; 282: 1737–1744.

Thase ME, Greenhouse JB, Frank E, Reynolds CF III, Pilkonis PA, Hurley K, Grochocinski V, Kupfer DJ. Treatment of major depression with psychotherapy or psychotherapy-pharmacotherapy combinations. Arch Gen Psychiatry 1997; 54: 1009–1015.

Ustun TB, Sartorius N (eds). Mental Illness in General Health Care: An International Study. London: John Wiley & Sons, 1995.

Ustun TB, Ayuso-Mateos JL, Chatterji S, Mathers C, Murray CJL. Global burden of depressive disorders in the year 2000. Br J Psychiatry 2004; 184: 386–392.

World Health Organization. The ICD-10 Classification of Mental and Behavioural Disorders: Diagnostic Criteria for Research. Geneva: World Health Organization, 1993.

# 5

# DIMENSIONS AND THE PSYCHOSIS PHENOTYPE

Judith Allardyce, M.B., Ch.B., MRCPsych, CCST

Trisha Suppes, M.D., Ph.D.

Jim van Os, M.D.

The current *Diagnostic and Statistical Manual of Mental Disorders,* Fourth Edition (DSM-IV; American Psychiatric Association 1994) classification of psychosis stems directly from the systematic clinical observations of Bleuler (1911/1950), Kraepelin (1919/1971), and Schneider (1959), who worked in the large asylums of Western Europe during the late nineteenth and early twentieth centuries. These institutions provided care for people with severe and debilitating conditions. There are at least two potentially important limitations to a classification system derived from such a selective case sample. First, because your clinical experience would be of severe cases in need of treatment, you would understandably conceptualize psychosis as a discrete disease entity, as a categorical construct, distinct from normality. This, however, may not reflect the true distribution of psychosis at the population level.

Second, the observed pattern of psychopathological co-occurrence may actually reflect symptoms, which are independent risk factors for hospital admission, becoming conditionally dependent in the institutional setting, a phenomenon known as Berkson's fallacy (bias). A community study has shown that positive and

Reprinted with permission from Allardyce J, Suppes T, van Os J. "Dimensions and the Psychosis Phenotype." *International Journal of Methods in Psychiatric Research* 2007; 16(S1): S34–S40.

negative symptoms are both independently associated with need for care (Maric et al. 2004). Such additive effects could inflate the positive/negative co-occurrence in hospital settings, indicating that the current conceptualization of schizophrenia as a unitary entity with high co-occurrence of positive and negative psychopathological domains may in part be the result of Berkson's bias.

Similar findings apply to the bipolar disorder construct. A general population study has demonstrated independent associations of manic and depressive symptoms, with need for care; while symptom co-occurrence was 17% in individuals known to services, it was only 7% in those not in the secondary health care system. These independent effects may well inflate depression/mania co-occurrence in institutional settings (Regeer et al., in press).

There is no doubt that the work of Kraepelin, Bleuler, and Schneider, respectively (and the classification systems that evolved from their insights), has greatly facilitated the acquisition of the knowledge we now have about psychosis. However, the walls of the asylum confined their observations, perhaps obscuring the true nature of the psychosis phenotype.

# Distribution of Psychosis in the General Population

The clinical definitions of psychosis may represent only a minor, possibly biased sample of the total psychosis phenotype present in the general population. This is consistent with the prevailing view that psychosis has a multifactorial etiology (similar to that seen in other chronic disorders such as diabetes and cardiovascular disease) where many different genes, which are neither necessary or sufficient causes, and of small effect, interact with each other and with environmental risk factors (Jones and Cannon 1998). It can be shown that such different combinations of risk factors must result in a gradation of exposure and an associated range of different expressions from normal through to clinical psychosis (continuum hypothesis). Mounting support for the continuum hypothesis comes from studies examining (1) the distribution of psychotic symptoms and psychotic proneness in the general population; (2) the pattern of genetic and non-genetic risk factor profiles in non-clinical and clinical samples; and (3) the transition from subclinical to clinical states over time (up to 25% in the largest prospective study to date [Poulton et al. 2000]).

The positive symptoms of psychosis, delusions, and hallucinations seem to have a continuous distribution in the general population (Eaton et al. 1991; Janssen et al. 2003; Johns et al. 2004; Kendler et al. 1996; King et al. 2005; Olfson et al. 2002; Peters et al. 1999; Poulton et al. 2000; Spauwen et al. 2003; Tien 1991; van Os et al. 2000b, 2001; Verdoux et al. 1998; Wiles et al. 2006). Prevalence estimates, in non-clinical samples, range from 4% (Eaton et al. 1991) to 17.5% (van

Os et al. 2000b) (with methodological differences likely to explain much of this variability). High rates do not appear to be secondary to measurement error due to self-report interview techniques, as high rates are also reported using non-self-report interviews by clinicians (Poulton et al. 2000; Spauwen et al. 2003). These rates also are not a reflection of unidentified cases "hidden" in the community, as only a very small proportion of those reporting positive psychotic symptoms fulfilled diagnostic criteria for DSM non-affective psychosis (Kendler et al. 1996; van Os et al. 2000b). That the psychosis phenotype is much more prevalent than previously thought is also supported by recent work showing that the lifetime prevalence of psychotic disorder, when multiple sources are taken into account, exceeds 3%, much higher than the traditional 0.6% (Perala et al. 2007). Studies of schizotypy (a personality trait characterized by a proneness to psychotic-like experiences) suggest that it is a quantitative rather than a qualitative trait, on a continuum from normality, through eccentricity, different combinations of schizotypal characteristics, to florid psychosis. Factor analyses of schizotypy extract three or possibly four dimensions: aberrant perceptions and beliefs, introvert/anhedonia, and conceptual disorganization (a factor solution some consider to be similar to that found in schizophrenia). This work suggests that psychosis proneness is a multidimensional continuous construct (Gruzelier 1996; Mata et al. 2003; Vollema and van den Bosch 1995).

Mood disturbance similarly appears to have a continuous distribution in the general population. Subthreshold depression and (hypo)mania, defined as the experience of distinct periods of depressive or (hypo)manic symptoms that do not fulfill the DSM-III-R (American Psychiatric Association 1987)/DSM-IV diagnostic criteria, appear to be common (Angst and Gamma 2002; Cuijpers et al. 2004), with prevalence rates of up to 13% for depression and 9% for hypomania (Angst and Merikangas 1997; Angst et al. 2003).

Evidence from longitudinal and cross-sectional studies of risk factors in general support a continuity of risk profiles for subclinical and clinical psychosis (Chapman et al. 1994; Kwapil et al. 1997; Peters et al. 1999; van Os et al. 2000b, 2001; Verdoux et al. 1998). However, one study has demonstrated some differences that will require further evaluation. Partly, these differences may be due to study design; for example, the study measured the effect of current urban residence on psychotic symptoms in elderly individuals who are likely to have moved many times and are at very low risk of developing incident psychotic symptoms, rather than studying urban birth/upbringing in young individuals who are most at risk for psychotic symptoms (Wiles et al. 2006).

Finally, longitudinal studies suggest that clinical psychosis emerges, from the pool of those with psychotic-like features, with a much higher than expected frequency (Bebbington and Nayani 1995; Chapman et al. 1994; Hanssen et al. 2005; Poulton et al. 2000). Non-clinical manic symptoms also appear to represent risk indicators for future clinical manic episodes (Regeer et al. 2006). Interestingly, the probability of developing incident bipolar disorder is substantially higher (approximately 7%) in individuals with both subclinical manic and psychotic symptoms (Kaymaz et al. 2006).

These studies suggest that both manic and psychosis phenotypes occur as part of a continuum from normality through to full-blown clinical disorders; that is, they are fundamentally dimensional in nature.

Superimposing categorical diagnoses onto latent continuous constructs results in loss of information, but this practice may yield useful shorthand approximations to facilitate communication among clinicians. Potential problems arise, however, if the categories are arbitrary or generated from samples with selection bias (e.g., from the severe end of the spectrum or institutional settings), where they potentially "misrepresent" the underlying patho-etiology. This is likely to impede our further understanding of the causes and correlates of psychosis. It may in part explain the current lack of replicable findings in the genetic and biological study of schizophrenia and bipolar disorder.

It is important to keep in mind that although a continuum of psychosis and bipolarity may exist, the diagnosis of need for care and the decision to treat always will remain dichotomous. Need for care results from the interaction between continuous phenotype and the person in terms of, for example, coping, social support, and the level of comorbid developmental impairment.

## Clinical Psychosis: Discrete Category or Psychopathological Dimensions?

Categories of psychoses defined in DSM-IV reflect historical notions of severe mental illness observed in institutionalized clinical settings. As discussed earlier, such settings may inflate the co-occurrence of symptoms, obscuring their true latent nature and generating spurious categories. The different psychotic diagnoses overlap in their pre-morbid risk factors, clinical presentations, management needs, and outcomes (Murray et al. 2004). This lack of discrimination casts doubt as to how clinically useful the categorical classification systems used today are (McGorry et al. 1998; Toomey et al. 1997) and has resulted in a search for alternative representations of psychoses. One approach is to identify psychopathological dimensions (groups of symptoms that occur together more often than would be expected by chance alone) using exploratory factor analyses. Individuals can then be defined by how high or low they score on the different dimensions, which may co-exist. The initial work in this area examined the factor structure of the diagnostic category of schizophrenia and found evidence for a three-factor solution (Bilder et al. 1985; Liddle 1987, 1992; Peralta et al. 1992), extracting positive, negative, and disorganized factors. The disorganization factor is the most unstable and least replicable of the three dimensions. However, a two-factor solution does not adequately represent the symptom correlations (Peralta et al. 1994), and the three-factor solution may in fact represent higher order factors of many more first-order dimensions (Peralta and Cuesta 1999). A five-factor solution with additional manic and depressive dimensions is found when measures of affective symptoms are included (Lindenmayer et al. 2004). When samples are expanded to include the full spectrum of psychoses, broadly similar five-factor solutions are found (Dikeos et al. 2006; Kitamura et al. 1995; Lindenmayer et al. 2004; McGorry et al. 1998; McIntosh et al. 2001; Murray et al. 2005; Ratakonda et al. 1998; Serretti and Olgiati 2004; Serretti et al. 2001), though there may be conflation of the disorganized and negative dimensions, especially in first-onset samples (McGorry et al. 1998). It seems that the dimensions generated from established cases of psychosis provide reasonably replicable, stable solutions in a variety of settings, diagnostic groups, and patient samples; however, the factor structure may be less stable around the time of presentation (Drake et al. 2003).

## THE CLINICAL VALIDITY OF DIMENSIONAL REPRESENTATIONS OF PSYCHOSIS

Nosological constructs such as psychopathological dimensions should be useful, that is, provide non-trivial information about course, outcome, and likely treatment response (Kendell 1989). A number of studies have examined the association of psychopathological dimensions with various clinically significant characteristics. The most consistent finding is a strong association of the negative dimension with indicators of poor (chronic deteriorating) course (Dikeos et al. 2006; Hollis 2000; Marengo et al. 2000; van Os et al. 1996; Wickham et al. 2001). The disorganization factor also predicts poor outcome, but this is a weaker and less consistent finding. The associations of other dimensions are inconsistent and markedly attenuated after adjustment for diagnosis (Dikeos et al. 2006).

A more informative method of assessing the usefulness of the dimensional approach is to compare the relative contribution of the dimensional factor scores and diagnostic categories in predicting the variability of clinically significant characteristics. Such studies consistently show the dimensional representations to be more useful at predicting clinical course and treatment needs, though the difference in the discriminative power may be rather small (Dikeos et al. 2006; Peralta et al. 2002; Rosenman et al. 2003; van Os et al. 1996).

One study has shown that while factor scores add to the predictive power of the diagnostic categories, the diagnostic categories did not increase the predictive power of the dimensional scores. This seems to suggest that the current diagnoses may partition symptom dimensions appropriately. However, models using both categorical and dimensional representations have better discriminative validity, suggesting that the most powerful approach to classification is the complementary use of both categorical diagnoses and dimensional scores (Dikeos et al. 2006).

## Practical Example

The following clinical example illustrates how concomitant categorical and dimensional assessment may facilitate patient care. A 45-year-old man with a 20-year history of bipolar I disorder presents with mild hypomanic symptoms: reduced need for sleep (2–3 hours less than usual per night), bright and cheerful affect, increased energy, and subjectively feels very productive at work. He has worked as an insurance agent manager of a large company for 10 years, where he is regarded as a conscientious, focused, calm, and task-oriented employee. At interview, he describes plans to reorganize the branch and carry this model throughout the company. This expansive but mild grandiosity does not meet criteria for delusional thinking but may be on a continuum with delusional grandiose thought. Use of a dimensional measurement would alert the clinician to offer appropriate intervention to avert manic relapse, which, if unmanaged, would escalate over a few days. His thought content would move to not only changing his branch, but also going to the head office to tell them how to run the company and telling them he should be CEO. This is one example for the mood case of mania. Similar examples could readily be drawn for patients diagnosed with schizophrenia, mania, or depression.

## Potential Limitations of a Dimensional Approach

To date, with different studies suggesting different numbers of factors or variations in factor composition, there is no definitive model for the symptom dimensions of psychosis, though the five-factor model comprising positive, negative, disorganized, manic, and depression dimensions is increasingly being considered to have internal validity. Most exploratory factor analytical studies have used chronic or mixed stage samples, however; if there are psychopathological changes during the course of a disorder (Eaton et al. 1995; Fenton and McGlashan 1991; Peralta and Cuesta 2001), samples with different distributions of "stage of disorder" will yield different symptom dimensions depending on the dominant stage studied. For example, there is no study in the current literature examining the predictive validity of symptom dimensions in first-episode cases of psychosis.

The current diagnostic categories facilitate diagnostic agreement (reliability) and communication among practitioners (Kendell and Jablensky 2003), and it may be that the introduction of dimensional measures could threaten this. However, what is being proposed initially is a dimensional measure that will complement the categorical diagnosis, perhaps generated from rating scales known to have relatively high inter-rater agreement—for example, the Positive and Negative Syndrome Scale (PANSS; Kay et al. 1987). Symptom-rating scales are now used routinely in clinical settings to monitor treatment response and relapse and to assess remission. The introduction of a formal dimensional measure in the classification system would, hopefully, coordinate and optimize this use.

It is important to decide over which diagnostic categories we measure any proposed psychotic dimensions. The revised classification system could be organized around the presence/absence of psychosis. However, it is quite possible that psychotic symptoms are not fundamental core features of the underlying diseases but, rather, are non-specific, perhaps even end-stage manifestations of a number of different pathological processes (Goldman-Rakic 1995). Crow (1990) has suggested that there exists an etiopathological continuum across schizophrenia, schizoaffective disorder, and affective illness, and a recent study of patients with psychotic and non-psychotic bipolar disorder and schizophrenia found a specific association between neuregulin 1 core-at-risk haplotype and "manic" forms of schizophrenia and "bipolar" forms of schizophrenia, supporting a biological continuum (Green et al. 2005). The literature suggests that substantial "hidden bipolarity" would be found in patients with unipolar depression if a mania dimension were additionally scored in the course of the diagnostic process (Benazzi and Akiskal 2003; Cassano et al. 2004), and negative symptoms have been demonstrated in patients with bipolar disorder (van Os et al. 2000a). The flexible scoring of dimensions across all psychotic and major affective disorders potentially could be more informative than a system where categorical diagnoses are kept artificially dimension-specific.

## Conclusions and Recommendations

It is essential that we understand how the psychosis phenotype or phenotypes exist in nature in order to study their determinants and outcomes. Further elucidation is likely to come from studies using descriptive and latent variable methodologies to identify fundamental categorical subtypes and/or continuous dimensions of psychopathology. In the future, it is likely these descriptive approaches will be complemented by the inclusion of putative etiological or pathophysiological indicators.

An ever-increasing number of published studies continue to examine dimensional approaches in schizophrenia and bipolar disorder. Dimensions are not diagnosis-specific, yet current categorical diagnoses require dimensional specificity. In the psychosis literature, affective and non-affective dimensions have been identified in people with psychosis, whereas in individuals with major mood syndromes, psychotic versus non-psychotic domains have been studied. A more productive approach may be to study dimensionality across all mood and psychotic syndromes.

The current evidence supports the complementary use of both categorical and dimensional representations of psychosis. Diagnostic models using both categorical diagnoses and dimensions have better predictive validity than either model independently, and flexible scoring of dimensions across all patients with psychotic and major affective disorders is likely to be especially informative.

# References

American Psychiatric Association. Diagnostic and Statistical Manual of Mental Disorders, 3rd Edition, Revised. Washington, DC: American Psychiatric Association, 1987

American Psychiatric Association. Diagnostic and Statistical Manual of Mental Disorders, 4th Edition. Washington, DC: American Psychiatric Association, 1994

Angst J, Gamma A. A new bipolar spectrum concept: a brief review. Bipolar Disord 2002; Suppl 1: 11–14.

Angst J, Merikangas K. The depressive spectrum: diagnostic classification and course. J Affect Disord 1997; 45(1– 2): 31–39, discussion 39–40.

Angst J, Gamma A, Benazzi F, Ajdacic V, Eich D, Rossler W. Toward a re-definition of subthreshold bipolarity: epidemiology and proposed criteria for bipolar-II, minor bipolar disorders and hypomania. J Affective Disorders 2003; 732: 133–146.

Bebbington P, Nayani T. The Psychosis Screening Questionnaire. Int J Methods Psychiatr Res 1995; 5: 11–19.

Benazzi F, Akiskal HS. Refining the evaluation of bipolar II: beyond the strict SCID-CV guidelines for hypomania. J Affect Disord 2003; 73(1–2): 33–38.

Bilder RM, Mukherjee S, Rieder RO, Pandurangi AK. Symptomatic and neuropsychological components of defect states. Schizophr Bull 1985; 11(3): 409–419.

Bleuler E. Dementia Praecox or the Group of Schizophrenias, 1911 (translated by Zinkin J). New York: International Universities Press, 1950.

Cassano GB, Rucci P, Frank E, Fagiolini A, Dell'Osso L, Shear MK, Kupfer DJ. The mood spectrum in unipolar and bipolar disorder: arguments for a unitary approach. Am J Psychiatry 2004; 161(7): 1264–1269.

Chapman LJ, Chapman JP, Kwapil TR, Eckblad M, Zinser MC. Putatively psychosis-prone subjects 10 years later. J Abnorm Psychol 1994; 103(2): 171–183.

Crow TJ. The continuum of psychosis and its genetic origins. The sixty-fifth Maudsley lecture. Br J Psychiatry 1990; 156: 788–797.

Cuijpers P, de Graaf R, van Dorsselaer S. Minor depression: risk profiles, functional disability, health care use and risk of developing major depression. J Affect Disord 2004; 79(1–3): 71–79.

Dikeos DGM, Wicham HMMF, McDonald CMMP, Walshe MB, Sigmundsson TM, Bramon EM, Grech AM, Touloupoulou TBMP, Murray RM, Sham PCM. Distribution of symptom dimensions across Kraepelinian divisions. Br J Psychiatry 2006; 189: 346–353.

Drake RJ, Dunn G, Tarrier N, Haddock G, Haley C, Lewis S. The evolution of symptoms in the early course of non-affective psychosis. Schizophr Res 2003; 63: 171–179.

Eaton WW, Romanoski A, Anthony JC, Nestadt G. Screening for psychosis in the general population with a self-report interview. J Nerv Ment Dis 1991; 179(11): 689–693.

Eaton WW, Thara R, Federman B, Melton B, Liang KY. Structure and course of positive and negative symptoms in schizophrenia. Arch Gen Psychiatry 1995; 52: 127–134.

Fenton WS, McGlashan TH. Natural history of schizophrenia subtypes. II. Positive and negative symptoms and long-term course. Arch Gen Psychiatry 1991; 48(11): 978–986.

Goldman-Rakic PS. More clues on "latent" schizophrenia point to developmental origins. Am J Psychiatry 1995; 152: 1701–1703.

Green EK, Raybould R, Macgregor S, Gordon-Smith K, Heron J, Hyde S, Grozeva D, Hamshere M, Williams N, Owen MJ, O'Donovan MC, Jones L, Jones I, Kirov G, Craddock N. Operation of the schizophrenia susceptibility gene, neuregulin 1, across traditional diagnostic boundaries to increase risk for bipolar disorder. Arch Gen Psychiatry 2005; 62(6): 642–648.

Gruzelier JH. The factorial structure of schizotypy: Part I. Affinities with syndromes of schizophrenia. Schizophr Bull 1996; 22(4): 611–620.

Hanssen M, Bak M, Bijl R, Vollebergh W, van Os J. The incidence and outcome of subclinical psychotic experiences in the general population. Br J Clin Psychol 2005; 44(Part 2): 181–191.

Hollis C. Adult outcomes of child- and adolescent-onset schizophrenia: diagnostic stability and predictive validity. Am J Psychiatry 2000; 157(10): 1652–1659.

Janssen I, Hanssen M, Bak M, Bijl RV, de Graaf R, Vollebergh W, McKenzie K, van Os J. Discrimination and delusional ideation. Br J Psychiatry 2003; 182: 71–76.

Johns LC, Cannon M, Singleton N, Murray RM, Farrell M, Brugha T, Bebbington P, Jenkins R, Meltzer H. Prevalence and correlates of self-reported psychotic symptoms in the British population. Br J Psychiatry 2004; 185: 298–305.

Jones P, Cannon M. The new epidemiology of schizophrenia. Psychiatr Clin North Am 1998; 21: 1–25.

Kay SR, Fiszbein A, Opler LA. The Positive and Negative Syndrome Scale (PANSS) for schizophrenia. Schizophr Bull 1987; 13(2): 261–276.

Kaymaz N, van Os J, de Graaf R, Ten Have M, Nolen W, Krabbendam L. The impact of subclinical psychosis on the transition from subclinical mania to bipolar disorder. J Affect Disord 2006; 98(1–2): 55–64.

Kendell R, Jablensky A. Distinguishing between the validity and the utility of psychiatric diagnoses. Am J Psychiatry 2003; 160: 4–12.

Kendell RE. Clinical validity. Psychol Med 1989; 471: 45–55.

Kendler KS, Gallagher TJ, Abelson JM, Kessler RC. Lifetime prevalence, demographic risk factors, and diagnostic validity of nonaffective psychosis as assessed in a U.S. community sample. The National Comorbidity Survey. Arch Gen Psychiatry 1996; 53(11): 1022–1031.

King M, Nazroo J, Weich S, McKenzie K, Bhui K, Karlsen S, Stansfeld S, Tyrer P, Blanchard M, Lloyd K, McManus S, Sproston K, Erens B. Psychotic symptoms in the general population of England—a comparison of ethnic groups (the EMPIRIC study). Soc Psychiatry Psychiatr Epidemiol 2005; 40(5): 375–381.

Kitamura T, Okazaki Y, Fujinawa A, Yoshino M, Kasahara Y. Symptoms of psychoses. A factor-analytic study. Br J Psychiatry 1995; 166: 236–240.

Kraepelin E. Dementia Praecox and Paraphrenia, 1919 (translated by Barkley RM). New York: Robert E Kreiger, 1971.

Kwapil TR, Miller MB, Zinser MC, Chapman J, Chapman LJ. Magical ideation and social anhedonia as predictors of psychosis proneness: a partial replication. J Abnorm Psychol 1997; 106(3): 491–495.

Liddle PF. The symptoms of chronic schizophrenia. A re-examination of positive-negative dichotomy. Br J Psychiatry 1987; 151: 145–151.

Liddle PF. Syndromes of schizophrenia on factor analysis (letter). Br J Psychiatry 1992; 161: 861.

Lindenmayer JP, Brown E, Baker RW, Schuh LM, Shao L, Tohen M, Ahmed S, Stauffer VL. An excitement subscale of the Positive and Negative Syndrome Scale. Schizophr Res 2004; 68: 331–337.

Marengo J, Harrow M, Herbener ES, Sands J. A prospective longitudinal 10-year study of schizophrenia's three major factors and depression. Psychiatry Res 2000; 97(1): 61–77.

Maric N, Myin-Germeys I, Delespaul P, de Graaf R, Vollebergh W, van Os J. Is our concept of schizophrenia influenced by Berkson's bias? Soc Psychiatry Psychiatr Epidemiol 2004; 39(8): 600–605.

Mata I, Gilvarry CM, Jones PB, Lewis SW, Murray RM, Sham PC. Schizotypal personality traits in nonpsychotic relatives are associated with positive symptoms in psychotic probands. Schizophr Bull 2003; 29(2): 273–283.

McGorry PD, Bell RC, Dudgeon PL, Jackson HJ. The dimensional structure of first episode psychosis: an exploratory factor analysis. Psychol Med 1998; 28: 935–947.

McIntosh AM, Forrester A, Lawrie SM, Byrne M, Harper A, Kestelman JN, Best JJ, Johnstone EC, Owens DG. A factor model of the functional psychoses and the relationship of factors to clinical variables and brain morphology. Psychol Med 2001; 31: 159–171.

Murray RM, Sham P, van Os J, Zanelli J, Cannon M, McDonald C. A developmental model for similarities and dissimilarities between schizophrenia and bipolar disorder. Schizophr Res 2004; 71(2–3): 405–416.

Murray V, McKee I, Miller PM, Young D, Muir WJ, Pelosi AJ, Blackwood DH. Dimensions and classes of psychosis in a population cohort: a four-class, four-dimension model of schizophrenia and affective psychoses. Psychol Med 2005; 35(4): 499–510.

Olfson M, Lewis-Fernandez R, Weissman MM, Feder A, Gameroff MJ, Pilowsky D, Fuentes M. Psychotic symptoms in an urban general medicine practice. Am J Psychiatry 2002; 159(8): 1412–1419.

Perala J, Suvisaari J, Saarni SI, Kuoppasalmi K, Isometsa E, Pirkola S, Partonen T, Tuulio-Henriksson A, Hintikka J, Kieseppa T, Harkanen T, Koskinen S, Lonnqvist J. Lifetime prevalence of psychotic and bipolar I disorders in a general population. Arch Gen Psychiatry 2007; 64: 19–28.

Peralta V, Cuesta MJ. Dimensional structure of psychotic symptoms: an item-level analysis of SAPS and SANS symptoms in psychotic disorders. Schizophr Res 1999; 38(1): 13–26.

Peralta V, Cuesta MJ. How many and which are the psychopathological dimensions in schizophrenia? issues influencing their ascertainment. Schizophr Res 2001; 49(3): 269–285.

Peralta V, de Leon J, Cuesta MJ. Are there more than two syndromes in schizophrenia? a critique of the positive-negative dichotomy [see comment]. Br J Psychiatry 1992; 161: 335–343.

Peralta V, Cuesta MJ, de Leon J. An empirical analysis of latent structures underlying schizophrenic symptoms: a four-syndrome model. Biol Psychiatry 1994; 36: 726–736.

Peralta V, Cuesta MJ, Giraldo C, Cardenas A, Gonzalez F. Classifying psychotic disorders: issues regarding categorical vs. dimensional approaches and time frame to assess symptoms. Eur Arch Psychiatry Clin Neurosci 2002; 252(1): 12–18.

Peters ER, Joseph SA, Garety PA. Measurement of delusional ideation in the normal population: introducing the PDI (Peters et al. Delusions Inventory). Schizophr Bull 1999; 25(3): 553–576.

Poulton R, Caspi A, Moffitt TE, Cannon M, Murray R, Harrington H. Children's self-reported psychotic symptoms and adult schizophreniform disorder: a 15-year longitudinal study. Arch Gen Psychiatry 2000; 57(11): 1053–1058.

Ratakonda S, Gorman JM, Yale SA, Amador XF. Characterization of psychotic conditions. Use of the domains of psychopathology model. Arch Gen Psychiatry 1998; 55: 75–81.

Regeer EJ, Krabbendam L, de Graaf R, ten Have M, Nolen WA, van Os J. A prospective study of the transition rates of subthreshold (hypo)mania and depression in the general population. Psychol Med 2006; 36: 619–627.

Regeer E, Krabbendam L, ten Have M, Nolen WA, van Os J. Berkson's bias and the mood dimensions of bipolar disorder. Soc Psychiatry Psychiatr Epidemiol (in press).

Rosenman S, Korten A, Medway J, Evans M. Dimensional vs. categorical diagnosis in psychosis. Acta Psychiatr Scand 2003; 107: 378–384.

Schneider K. Clinical Psychopathology. New York: Grune & Stratton, 1959.

Serretti A, Olgiati P. Dimensions of major psychoses: a confirmatory factor analysis of six competing models. Psychiatry Res 2004; 127: 101–109.

Serretti A, Rietschel M, Lattuada E, Krauss H, Schulze TG, Muller DJ, Maier W, Smeraldi E. Major psychoses symptomatology: factor analysis of 2241 psychotic subjects. Eur Arch Psychiatry Clin Neurosci 2001; 251: 193–198.

Spauwen J, Krabbendam L, Lieb R, Wittchen HU, van Os J. Sex differences in psychosis: normal or pathological? Schizophr Res 2003; 62: 45–49.

Tien AY. Distributions of hallucinations in the population. Soc Psychiatry Psychiatr Epidemiol 1991; 26(6): 287–292.

Toomey R, Kremen WS, Simpson JC, Samson JA, Seidman LJ, Lyons MJ, Faraone SV, Tsuang MT. Revisiting the factor structure for positive and negative symptoms: evidence from a large heterogeneous group of psychiatric patients. Am J Psychiatry 1997; 154: 371–377.

van Os J, Fahy TA, Jones P, Harvey I, Sham P, Lewis S, Bebbington P, Toone B, Williams M, Murray R. Psychopathological syndromes in the functional psychoses: associations with course and outcome. Psychol Med 1996; 26: 161–176.

van Os J, Gilvarry C, Bale R, van Horn E, Tattan T, White I, Murray R. Diagnostic value of the DSM and ICD categories of psychosis: an evidence-based approach. UK700 Group. Soc Psychiatry Psychiatr Epidemiol 2000a; 35(7): 305–311.

van Os J, Hanssen M, Bijl RV, Ravelli A. Strauss (1969) revisited: a psychosis continuum in the general population? Schizophr Res 2000b; 45: 11–20.

van Os J, Hanssen M, Bijl RV, Vollebergh W. Prevalence of psychotic disorder and community level of psychotic symptoms: an urban-rural comparison. Arch Gen Psychiatry 2001; 58(7): 663–668.

Verdoux H, Maurice-Tison S, Gay B, van Os J, Salamon R, Bourgeois ML. A survey of delusional ideation in primary-care patients. Psychol Med 1998; 28(1): 127–134.

Vollema MG, van den Bosch RJ. The multidimensionality of schizotypy. Schizophr Bull 1995; 21(1): 19–31.

Wickham H, Walsh C, Asherson P, Taylor C, Sigmundson T, Gill M, Owen MJ, McGuffin P, Murray R, Sham P. Familiarity of symptom dimensions in schizophrenia. Schizophr Res 2001; 47(2–3): 223–232.

Wiles NJ, Zammit S, Bebbington P, Singleton N, Meltzer H, Lewis G. Self-reported psychotic symptoms in the general population: results from the longitudinal study of the British National Psychiatric Morbidity Survey. Br J Psychiatry 2006; 188: 519–526.

# 6

# SUPPLEMENTARY DIMENSIONAL ASSESSMENT IN ANXIETY DISORDERS

M. Katherine Shear, M.D.
Ingvar Bjelland, M.D., Ph.D.
Katja Beesdo, Ph.D.
Andrew T. Gloster, Ph.D.
Hans-Ulrich Wittchen, Ph.D.

The publication of the *Diagnostic and Statistical Manual of Mental Disorders,* Third Edition (DSM-III; American Psychiatric Association 1980) in 1980 marked the advent of a new era of conceptualizing phobic and anxiety disorders, previously assigned to a broader category of "neuroses" that included anxiety, phobic, and obsessive-compulsive neurosis. The revised diagnostic system grouped conditions sharing several common features of symptomatic anxiety into an anxiety disorders section, separate from depression and somatoform disorders. Within the anxiety disorders, explicit criteria are provided for individual diagnostic categories. The DSM-IV (American Psychiatric Association 1994) classification includes panic disorder with and without agoraphobia, agoraphobia without panic disorder, social phobia, specific phobia, obsessive-compulsive disorder (OCD), posttraumatic

Reprinted with permission from Shear MK, Bjelland I, Beesdo K, Gloster AT, Wittchen H-U. "Supplementary Dimensional Assessment in Anxiety Disorders." *International Journal of Methods in Psychiatric Research* 2007; 16(S1): S52–S64.

stress disorder (PTSD), acute stress disorder, and generalized anxiety disorder (GAD) within an overall section of anxiety disorders, though these conditions have many phenotypic differences. Noteworthy changes include (a) replacing anxiety neurosis with panic disorder and GAD, (b) partitioning phobic neuroses into agoraphobia, social phobia, and various types of specific phobia, and (c) including a new category of PTSD and, later, acute stress disorder. Further, adult anxiety disorder criteria were slightly modified to allow their application in childhood, suggesting developmental continuity of these conditions. Notably, though, separation anxiety disorder remained within the section of childhood disorders, with its extension into adulthood left ambiguous.

DSM-III introduced an atheoretical descriptive approach that employed well-specified diagnostic criteria and clearly defined algorithms. This greatly improved reliability and effective communication among mental health professionals. These changes facilitated development of improved diagnostic assessment instruments (e.g., Structured Clinical Interview for DSM [First and Gibbon 2004; Spitzer et al. 1992], Composite International Diagnostic Interview [World Health Organization 1990]) and were instrumental in the development and testing of efficacious treatments. Nonetheless, the new system also met considerable criticism.

Some challenged the justification for criteria used to define diagnostic thresholds and category boundaries, as well as decisions about core psychopathological components (Angst et al. 1997; Goldberg 1996). Others questioned the validity of the partitions among anxiety disorders and between anxiety and other disorders (Krueger 1999), arguing that the DSM approach leads to a good deal of artificial comorbidity. Still others questioned the appropriateness of the anxiety classification for children (see Hudziak et al., Chapter 8), as well as the elderly (Knäuper 1999). Designers of DSM-III, DSM-III-R (American Psychiatric Association 1987), and DSM-IV were aware of many of these problems. In the introduction to each edition, the committee noted that categorical criteria and thresholds were provisional and in need of empirical confirmation, validation, and/or modification (American Psychiatric Association 1980, 1987, 1994, 2000).

In this chapter we will describe some of the ways dimensional approaches have been used in anxiety disorders, make suggestions about the best way to integrate categorical and dimensional approaches, and provide suggestions for future research directions that could assist in developing the most appropriate dimensional strategies. It is important to bear in mind that there are different dimensional approaches in the anxiety literature, depending on the clinical or research objective of the investigator. For example, the term "dimensional" is used to refer to the use of continuous rather than categorical diagnostic criteria, to dimensional severity within a diagnostic category, to dimensions derived from higher order factor analytic approaches, to cross-cutting psychopathological dimensions like panic attacks, and to dimensions of developmental continuity. These different approaches to dimensional assessment reflect the many different purposes of diagnostic criteria.

A comprehensive review of all types of dimensional assessment in anxiety is beyond the scope of this chapter. Instead, we provide a selective review of the literature, focusing on three generic approaches to dimensional assessment: (a) continuous assessment of core diagnostic features of individual anxiety disorders, (b) dimensional assessment of facets of anxiety common to different DSM disorders, and other "cross-cutting" approaches, and (c) hybrid approaches, such as spectrum and higher order factor analytic approaches. Figure 6–1 depicts these concepts and highlights disorder-specific and cross-cutting assessment domains. We conclude by discussing how an integrated model that retains the current categorical system and includes cross-cutting dimensional assessments might be a productive direction in DSM-V anxiety disorders and by suggesting research directions that might inform decisions about whether and how to implement such a plan.

# Continuous Assessment Linked to Specific DSM-IV Disorders

Dimensional measures within diagnostic categories have a long and rich tradition in clinical, basic, and applied anxiety disorders research across the life span. Behavioral psychotherapists and pharmacotherapists regularly employ dimensional assessment to evaluate treatment results. As a result of decades of research, psychometrically sound dimensional assessment instruments are available for virtually any psychopathological domain relevant to anxiety disorders. There are instruments to assess any number of characteristics (e.g., cognitive-affective symptoms, avoidance behavior, etc.), including quantity, frequency, intensity, and/or severity. Many of these scales were developed for the purpose of planning and/or evaluating cognitive-behavioral therapy (CBT) treatments.

Some instruments used to rate psychopathology relevant to a specific diagnosis focus on a single symptom or functional domain, while others address several domains. Examples of unidimensional scales used to assess individuals with agoraphobia and/or panic disorder are the Mobility Inventory (MI; Chambless et al. 1985) and the Agoraphobic Cognitions Questionnaire (ACQ; Chambless et al. 1984). The MI rates the quantity and frequency of avoidance of different agoraphobic situations, whereas the ACQ assesses cognitive bias thought to be associated with physical symptoms of panic disorder. Similarly, the Fear of Negative Evaluation Scale (FNE; Watson and Friend 1969) rates intensity of cognitive symptoms thought to underlie social phobia. The Liebowitz Social Anxiety Scale (LSAS; Liebowitz 1987) rates fear and avoidance of social interaction and performance situations. Targeted, unidimensional scales have their place in clinical and research studies. They can be used to identify treatment mediators and/or moderators, to explore putative psychopathological processes within and across disorders, and to characterize residual symptoms. Scales such as these are often used by behavior therapists to guide and monitor treatment.

By anxiety diagnosis

Across diagnoses by domain

| DSM-IV anxiety diagnoses | Specific and shared evaluation domains* according to diagnostic criteria | | | | | | |
|---|---|---|---|---|---|---|---|
| | Diagnosis-specific features | Anxiety reaction/panic | Anticipatory anxiety | Avoidance behavior | Impairment, disability | Distress/negative affect | Duration, persistence |
| Panic disorder w/o agoraphobia | | | | | | | |
| Panic disorder with agoraphobia | | | | | | | |
| Agoraphobia w/o history of panic | | | | | | | |
| GAD | | | | | | | |
| Specific phobias | | | | | | | |
| Social phobia | | | | | | | |
| OCD | | | | | | | |
| PTSD | | | | | | | |
| Acute stress disorder | | | | | | | |
| Separation anxiety disorder | | | | | | | |

*Each domain can be rated continuously by severity, frequency, etc. Other possible domains may include etiological factors (neurobiological, developmental, etc.).

**FIGURE 6–1.** Diagnosis-specific and cross-cutting assessment domains of anxiety disorders.

*Note.* GAD=generalized anxiety disorder; OCD=obsessive-compulsive disorder; PTSD=posttraumatic stress disorder.

There are hundreds of unidimensional scales that can be used to supplement diagnostic assessments and can be useful for measuring change, estimating improvement, or exploring the processes of change. Most assess current but not lifetime symptoms. Importantly, few are useful in all clinical situations. Rather, their utility depends upon the clinical characteristics of the patient, the method of intervention, and specific goals of the individual treatment plan.

Multidimensional scales that rate the severity of criterion symptoms of different DSM-IV disorders have also been developed. The prototype for this kind of scale is the Yale-Brown Obsessive Compulsive Scale (Y-BOCS; Goodman et al. 1989). The Y-BOCS was designed to assess the severity of various facets (i.e., duration, resultant interference, associated distress, self-initiated resistance against symptoms, and degree of control over the symptoms) on a 0–4 scale of obsessions and compulsions, rated separately. The scale includes a checklist of over 50 common OCD symptoms that is used as a reference for the symptom ratings. This convention helps both the patient and interviewer to understand the nature of the symptom profile before rating symptom-related distress and interference.

Among a large group of studies of this instrument, factor analysis of the Y-BOCS yielded a two-factor structure, consisting of disturbance and severity (Amir et al. 1997). The Y-BOCS was designed to reflect treatment change and has become the gold standard for treatment studies of OCD as well as a model for the development of comparable measures for other disorders. The Panic Disorder Severity Scale (PDSS; Shear et al. 2001b) and Generalized Anxiety Disorder Severity Scale (GADSS; Shear et al. 2006) are other examples of this type of scale. The PDSS begins by defining panic attacks and rates the frequency and distress caused by panic and limited symptom episodes, severity of anticipatory anxiety, degree of sensation avoidance and agoraphobic avoidance, and degree of work/social impairment. The GADSS catalogues types of work and assesses symptom distress and impairment in GAD. These scales are convenient ways of obtaining a severity measure for use in treatment outcome. Importantly, these scales have not been developed by systematic psychometric methods but rather comprise a format for standard evaluation of the severity of DSM-IV criterion symptoms. In this, they resemble the DSM criteria themselves. Thus, while helpful for clinical purposes, and useful in epidemiological and other types of research studies, these scales do not provide criterion validation for diagnostic categories.

A different approach to dimensional assessment can be used to explore the validity of DSM diagnostic categories. Interestingly, although committees that developed DSM-III to DSM-IV called for systematic research into boundaries and thresholds, little systematic study has been undertaken to examine criteria validity, algorithm thresholds, or distinctiveness of symptoms across disorders. The possible exception is GAD. Studies of this disorder illustrate how research could be undertaken to test current categorical DSM criteria, develop dimensional variants, and suggest improved definitions for core symptoms, duration criteria, and associated features.

## EXCESSIVENESS VERSUS NON-EXCESSIVENESS OF WORRY IN GAD

DSM-IV criteria for GAD require that worrying be excessive, but available research suggests that GAD is not very different with or without excessive worry (Ruscio et al. 2005). There appears to be no difference in sociodemographic characteristics or family aggregation between GAD with and without excessive worry. Instead, degree of excessiveness appears to define a severity gradient, and GAD with persistent excessive worry is a more severe variant that begins earlier in life, has a more chronic course, and is associated with greater symptom severity and psychiatric comorbidity than GAD without excessive worry.

## GAD DURATION/PERSISTENCE CRITERIA

In DSM-III, GAD diagnosis required symptoms lasting at least 1 month. The duration was changed to 6 months in DSM-III-R and DSM-IV in an attempt to reduce the high rate of comorbidity found with the shorter duration. Systematic research into different durations revealed that the persistence criterion is poorly supported by research: Epidemiologic data indicate that GAD does occur in episodes with variable duration (Beesdo 2006; Grant et al. 2005) and that GAD cases with a maximum episode duration of 1–5 months do not differ greatly from those with episodes of 6 months or longer in terms of onset, persistence, impairment, comorbidity, parental GAD, or sociodemographic correlates (Kessler et al. 2005).

## GAD-ASSOCIATED SYMPTOMS

DSM-IV diagnostic criteria require three out of six associated symptoms to be present, in addition to worry, in order to diagnose GAD. However, a requirement for two rather than three of these symptoms has little effect on prevalence (Ruscio et al. 2006). Among adolescents and young adults with GAD, four to five out of the six symptoms are reported on average, with each symptom endorsed by at least 50% of the cases (Beesdo 2006). It is likely that the greater the number of GAD symptoms (beyond the one required by diagnosis), the greater the severity and impairment. A dimensional measure of GAD, such as the GADSS, could test this expectation. Discussions for DSM-V will need to take into consideration these findings for GAD and other anxiety disorders.

# Generic Dimensional and Other Cross-Cutting Approaches

A different approach to dimensional assessment crosses current diagnostic boundaries by rating symptoms common to multiple anxiety disorders. This approach highlights the fact that shared symptoms form the basis for grouping anxiety disorders into a single section of DSM-IV. Shared symptom domains are illustrated in Figure 6–1. In addition to providing an efficient method of assessment across anxiety disorders, this approach also provides a way of measuring severity of co-occurring anxiety symptomatology in other, non-anxiety disorders such as mood or psychotic disorders or substance abuse. For example, co-occurring anxiety symptoms have been found to be frequent and associated with different patterns of illness among depressed outpatients (Fava et al. 2006).

The best known examples of these scales are the Hamilton Anxiety Rating Scale (Ham-A; Hamilton 1959) and the Hospital Anxiety and Depression Scale (HADS; Zigmond and Snaith 1983). However, there are numerous other cross-cutting symptom scales. The Brief Psychiatric Rating Scale (BPRS; Overall and Gorman 1962) is a clinician-administered interview that assesses a broad range of symptoms, including items on anxiety. Examples of self-report questionnaires include the State-Trait Anxiety Inventory (STAI; Spielberger et al. 1970) and the Anxiety Sensitivity Index (ASI; Reiss et al. 1986). The STAI measures non-specific state and trait levels of anxiety. Respondents indicate how much each statement reflects how they feel right now, at this moment (state version), or how they generally feel (trait version) on four-point scales. The ASI measures the degree to which one believes anxiety and its symptoms will cause negative psychological, physiological, and social consequences. Interestingly, the ASI was originally conceptualized as a way of assessing the core fear in panic disorder but has since been associated with all anxiety disorders. The revised ASI (ASI-R; Taylor and Cox 1998) was derived to more thoroughly measure the construct of anxiety sensitivity. The value of these broad instruments as classificatory tools remains underinvestigated.

A recent development in dimensional assessment focuses on underlying constructs operating across different anxiety disorders. One such scale is based on the idea that for each anxiety disorder there is a pathological concern about threat and that symptoms can be conceptualized as lying on a threat-imminence continuum (Craske 1999, 2003). Informed by ethological research (Fanselow and Lester 1988), the developers of this concept hypothesize that anxiety symptoms are not constant but rather vary as a function of proximity to stimuli perceived as dangerous, with proximity evaluated across space, time, and intensity. The resulting responses range from anxious worry about a possible future threat to fear when facing a clear threat and panic when confronted with immediate danger. These responses serve different functions. On the distal end, worry about an uncertain threat serves to orient and plan for possible response. Some investigators claim that worry is an element of all anxiety disorders (Barlow 2002). On the other end of the continuum, panic generated in the immediate presence of a significant danger is associated with a fight/flight or freezing response. So conceived, the threat-imminence continuum provides a framework from which the presence of symptoms across different anxiety disorders can be understood. Studies showing that panic and worry occur among individuals who do not develop diagnosable anxiety disorders are consistent with the idea of a threat-imminence continuum. Conversely, this same observation raises the important question of why some individuals develop anxiety disorders while others with similar experiences do not.

Avoidance is common to all anxiety disorders. Excessive use of escape and avoidance as a response to threat may be a part of the answer to the question of why people develop DSM-IV anxiety disorders. Avoidance behaviors contribute importantly to functional impairment and can interfere with learning about the accuracy of perceived threat stimuli (e.g., Eifert and Forsyth 2005). It is important to note that avoidance occurs across both external and internal domains (e.g., avoidance of situations, activities, feelings, thoughts, memories), all of which serve the function of reducing exposure to a perceived threat. Avoidance limits encounters with potentially threatening experiences at the expense of the potential for satisfying activities. Overuse of avoidance limits the development of coping strategies for everyday life problems and interferes with emotional processing and correction of overestimation of threat. It is likely that a marked tendency for avoidance is an important mechanism for the onset and maintenance of pathological anxiety. Importantly, by the nature of avoidance, individuals often fail to report their avoidance behaviors spontaneously or with simple questions. The central role of avoidance across anxiety disorders and the need for detailed questioning make this an excellent candidate for dimensional assessment.

Panic attacks also occur across anxiety and other psychiatric disorders (Goodwin et al. 2004; Reed and Wittchen 1998). DSM-IV provides a definition of panic outside of any specific disorder, calling attention to the fact that panic can occur in association with any anxiety disorder and with other mental disorders. The decision to indicate that panic is cross-cutting has proved to be important, as there is now strong evidence that the occurrence of panic is a reliable marker for a range of clinically important problems, including higher illness severity, more suicidality, and lower treatment responsiveness (Bittner et al. 2004; Goodwin and Hamilton 2001; Goodwin and Roy-Byrne 2006; Wittchen et al. 2003). Placement of panic as a symptom defined separately and seen across disorders provides a beginning for inclusion of other cross-cutting anxiety symptoms.

The criteria of impairment and distress are elements of every DSM anxiety disorder. As with other DSM diagnoses, impairment and distress are not clearly defined in the manual. Numerous dimensional assessments of these criteria exist, however. For example, in pharmacotherapy studies impairment is frequently measured with the Sheehan Disability Scale (SDS; Sheehan 2000). Psychotherapy studies utilize the Work and Social Adjustment Scale (Mundt et al. 2002). These scales assess the patient's degree of disability via items evaluating impairment in work/school, social life/leisure activities, and family life/home responsibilities. Multiple other scales of this sort also exist, ranging from generic disability scales such as the World Health Organization Disability Assessment Schedule

(WHODAS; World Health Organization 2000) to full-blown interview approaches such as the Groningen Social Disabilities Schedule (GSDS; Wiersma et al. 1988, 1990). The performance of these scales among patients with anxiety disorders is currently untested.

# Hybrid Approaches: Spectrum Approach and Higher Order Categories

There is an additional group of diverse and conceptually heterogeneous "hybrid" dimensional approaches that propose alternative or reorganized classifications of disorders using various methods. Included among these are (1) higher order factors and (2) spectrum approaches.

## HIGHER ORDER APPROACHES

The first of these hybrid conceptualizations entails a reorganization of DSM in which mood and anxiety disorders are grouped together. Symptom overlap and high levels of comorbidity among the anxiety disorders and between anxiety and other disorders have stimulated research investigating the factor structure underlying these disorders in an effort to elucidate core psychopathological processes of phenotypic psychopathology. The tripartite model by Clark and colleagues (Clark and Watson 1991; D.A. Clark et al. 1994; L.A. Clark et al. 1994; Watson et al. 1995) postulates a three-component structure for anxiety and depressive syndromes: "general affective distress" or negative affect as unspecific component, "anhedonia" or the lack of positive affect as specific for depression, and "physiological hyperarousal" or somatic tension as specific for anxiety. A similar but hierarchical conceptualization was proposed by Barlow and colleagues (Barlow 1988, 1991; Barlow and Di Nardo 1991; Zinbarg and Barlow 1996). They suggest a higher order factor of "negative affect" that is common to both anxiety and depressive disorders. On a lower level, each anxiety disorder incorporates a specific factor. Based on a series of factor-analytic investigations, Krueger and others (Krueger 1999; Krueger et al. 1998; Vollebergh et al. 2001) proposed a higher order, "internalizing disorder" factor with two subfactors: "anxious-misery" (containing depressive disorders and GAD) and "fear" (containing phobias and panic disorders).

These different subtypes have some empirical support, however with considerable methodological and statistical constraints (Wittchen et al. 1999). The analyses are based on a priori categorical decisions usually from diagnostic interviews. Threshold issues, developmental stage, and age have received little attention. Further, only a limited number of DSM disorders were used for analyses, ignoring major diagnostic categories such as PTSD, OCD, or subtypes of phobias. Among methodological factors, subject homogeneity and varying statistical approaches must be viewed critically. Overall, clinical utility of this set of dimensional proposals is quite limited. However, others (Watson 2005; Widiger 2005; Widiger and Clark 2000; Widiger and Samuel 2005) call for a radical revision of DSM. We believe it is unwise and premature to draw strong conclusions and directions for diagnostic nomenclature from methodologically variable statistical studies. Doing so would create considerable confusion regarding the interpretation of a large body of intervention literature that clearly identifies efficacious treatments for existing categories. Moreover, data support both cross-cutting and specific domains of symptoms for mood and anxiety disorders. It is possible to develop cross-cutting higher order dimensional ratings relevant to mood and anxiety disorders without changing either the definition of DSM-IV disorders or the organization of the diagnostic manual. Implementation of this approach could be very useful for both clinicians and researchers.

## SPECTRUM APPROACHES

A second and very different hybrid approach posits that a spectrum of symptoms or syndromes emerges in different patterns from a core central pathology. Several spectrum approaches exist (e.g., Akiskal 2003; Hollander 2005; Lara et al. 2006), but that by Cassano and colleagues (discussed later) arguably represents the approach with the most empirical support. This group examines dimensional symptoms, behavioral traits, and response orientations associated with DSM-IV categorical disorders and defines a spectrum of criterion symptoms and non-criterion clinical features that emanate from each DSM-IV category.

The spectrum approach of Cassano and colleagues has developed and validated multiple assessment instruments for the anxiety disorders (e.g., Cassano et al. 1997; Frank et al. 1998). These instruments have been found to provide important information about a range of symptoms not currently included in DSM-IV that occur in association with specific DSM-IV disorders but can also comprise clinically meaningful comorbidity in other conditions. The Structured Clinical Interview for Panic-Agoraphobic Spectrum (SCI-PAS; Cassano et al. 1999) is one example of the spectrum approach to assessment. This instrument provides a lifetime appraisal of eight domains of clinical features: (1) separation sensitivity, (2) panic-like symptoms, (3) stress sensitivity, (4) medication and substance sensitivity, (5) anxious expectation, (6) agoraphobia, (7) illness phobia and hypochondriasis, and (8) reassurance orientation. The SCI-PAS has been shown to be a useful measure of a group of symptoms that are more likely to be present among patients with panic disorder than among other psychiatric patients and normal control subjects (Shear et al. 2001a). Further, studies conducted in the United States and Italy show similar spectrum profiles in Italian and American patients and control subjects (Frank et al. 2005). Moreover, studies have shown that the presence of panic spectrum comorbidity, in the absence of DSM-IV panic disorder, is an important predictor of outcome among patients with major depression (Frank et al. 2002b) and bipolar disorder (Frank et al. 2002a). Spectrum instruments could be used in genetic and neurobiological studies (e.g., Martini et al. 2004). The occurrence of clinically significant spectrum symptoms in the absence of DSM-IV disorders may provide a view of psychopathology that would otherwise be missed (e.g., Manfredini et al. 2005). These findings support the idea that this hybrid categorical-dimensional model has the potential to be clinically useful and to contribute to a better understanding of symptom domains that cross current diagnostic categories.

# Future Research Needs and Conclusions

In summary, our selected review of dimensional assessment approaches in anxiety disorders illustrates how symptom domains described by DSM-IV anxiety disorders can be measured with continuous measures. Dimensional approaches can be disorder-focused, cross-cutting, or hybrid models. In fact, dimensional measures of all three types have been widely used in anxiety disorder research for decades. Recent authors advocate for their routine use in clinical practice as a tool for measurement-based care (Trivedi et al. 2006). It is clear that dimensional assessment can enrich our understanding of anxiety in a variety of ways and that the best approach would be dictated by the question or concern being addressed. Examples of different purposes of diagnostic assessment include determining whether an individual has sufficient distress and/or impairment to profit from treatment; monitoring the progress of treatment; doing genetic, neurobiological, developmental, and other mechanisms studies; determining developmental course of different disorders; examining the epidemiological distribution of different conditions and their severity in the community; exploring rates and significance of co-occurrence of disorders to determine effects on course or treatment outcome; and collecting data that will help discover new subtype distinctions or diagnostic boundary distinctions.

Given the varied needs associated with different kinds of studies and clinical activities, we strongly believe that the field needs to continue to utilize the categorical approaches best suited to specific objectives. However, as we consider revisions to DSM-IV, we must revisit the question as to what degree supplementary dimensional approaches should be incorporated. Given the extensive information now available for anxiety disorders, selectively reviewed in this chapter, we assert that it is time to seriously consider the addition of dimensional assessment in DSM-V. Keeping in mind that diagnosis is used for many purposes, we believe that the most useful approach would be to add cross-cutting anxiety assessments to the existing categorical system. This strategy has a precedent in the placement of panic attacks in DSM-IV.

There is a panoply of dimensional measures of anxiety-related constructs, with literally thousands of validated scales available to assess different domains of anxiety symptoms. The question of which ones should be considered standard and potentially included in DSM-V is a daunting one. Data collected by researchers differ depending upon the orientation (i.e., psychology versus psychiatry) and goals of a given investigator's research program and those of each specific project. The analytic strategy chosen for a particular study or group of studies is based on specific assumptions. Assumptions differ across projects, and these differences lead to different types of conclusions independent of the phenomenon of interest (e.g., cluster analysis, latent class analyses, and factor analysis are specifically designed to detect subgroups of like items, people, etc.). Most importantly, many of these differences are based on different purposes of symptom assessment across studies, research centers, and disciplines. Therefore, the dimensional approach we advocate is based on our view of the main purpose of the diagnostic manual. We reiterate that we do not mean to suggest that this is the best approach for all purposes.

There is growing agreement that there are both shared and discrete symptoms among anxiety disorders and between mood and anxiety disorders (Fergusson et al. 2006; Gregory et al. 2007). More research is needed to clarify which are shared and which are symptoms specific to each condition, and how these should be best represented in a diagnostic system. We suggest that DSM include both rows and columns as outlined in Figure 6–1. In particular, we advocate the inclusion of anticipatory anxiety, phobic symptoms, and anxiety-related impairment and distress, along with panic attacks as cross-cutting symptoms. This approach could be useful in a number of ways. We discuss two of them here.

First, there is a need to define and measure the core symptom domains shared by all anxiety disorders in the same way and consistently. This approach has already proved highly useful with panic symptoms, both across anxiety disorders and within other DSM-IV disorders. There is growing evidence for the importance of avoidance in the onset and maintenance of clinically significant anxiety. Moreover, according to the threat-imminence model, avoidance may be fueled by anticipatory anxiety and worry. Measuring these constructs across disorders could provide important insights into these various facets of anxiety and might also provide better information for genetic studies, developmental studies, epidemiology, and treatment studies. Cross-cutting measures could also be useful to clinicians who are interested in deciding whom to treat and in monitoring the effects of their treatment.

Secondly, an integrated model including current DSM-IV disorders as well as cross-cutting dimensional measures could be used as a device for illness staging (see Figure 6–2). Such staging might entail a developmental perspective and/or an illness course characterization.

Since Donald Klein's (1981) groundbreaking work on panic staging, there has been considerable interest in this type of developmental approach. Lack of standardized assessment of cross-cutting constructs such as avoidance has impeded the validation of such progression, yet there is indirect support for this model from

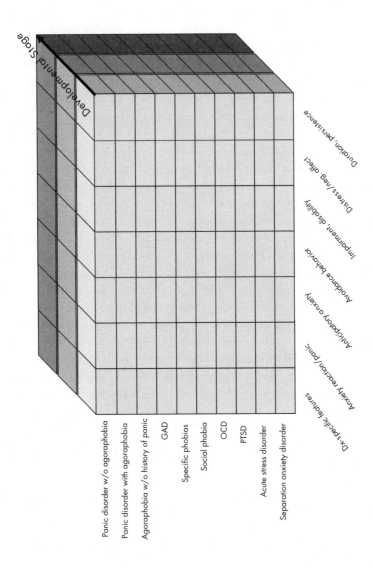

**FIGURE 6–2.** Diagnostic domains by development stage.

*Note.* Dx=diagnosis; neg.=negative.

prospective-longitudinal studies. Evidence from these studies further indicates that the occurrence of panic attacks is a sensitive marker for emerging severe psychopathology across disorders. The Early Developmental Stages of Psychopathology (EDSP) study found that over 90% of subjects with a panic attack go on to eventually develop a full-blown DSM-IV anxiety, affective, or other mental disorder (Goodwin et al. 2004; Reed and Wittchen 1998). This suggests that panic attacks, although a core feature of panic disorder, might be a severity marker across diagnoses. We need to know if this is also the case for other facets of anxiety.

Staging approaches have a long tradition in internal medicine and have been found to be clinically useful. For example, staging is used in diabetes mellitus and its micro- and macrovascular complications (Haffner 2006). We believe a staging approach could also be fruitfully developed and used in clinical work with individuals with mental disorders. Such an approach might be helpful in defining illness course and treatment needs. For example, an individual with stage I symptoms might be someone for whom psychoeducation and watchful waiting would be appropriate. For stage II, a monotherapy might be appropriate, while for stage III (or IV), combined treatment might be indicated. Figures 6–2 and 6–3 illustrate different ways such a model might be applicable across anxiety disorders and over the life span. For example, a recent study identified a developmental pathway in which specific phobias in childhood appear to be precursors for more severe complications in adulthood (Emmelkamp and Wittchen, in press).

To conclude, we believe that replacing categorical diagnostic criteria with dimensional assessment would not serve the field well at this point in time. The current DSM structure for anxiety disorder should be preserved, since it supplies simple, reliable rules for categorical assignments required for clinical and research purposes. This system provides the link to a very large body of important and useful empirical data. However, extending the idea of cross-cutting symptoms among the different anxiety disorders and across the wider diagnostic groups could also be helpful in learning more about which symptoms are shared and which are diagnostically different. It may be useful to incorporate several of the established dimensional assessments as a supplement to existing diagnostic procedures. Additionally, from a developmental perspective and in terms of treatment planning, we suggest adoption of a developmental staging method, as such an assessment may help clinicians and researchers as they strive to understand, plan treatments, and evaluate outcome.

# References

Akiskal HS. Validating "hard" and "soft" phenotypes within the bipolar spectrum: continuity or discontinuity? J Affect Disord 2003; 73: 1–5.

American Psychiatric Association. Diagnostic and Statistical Manual of Mental Disorders, 3rd Edition. Washington, DC: American Psychiatric Association, 1980.

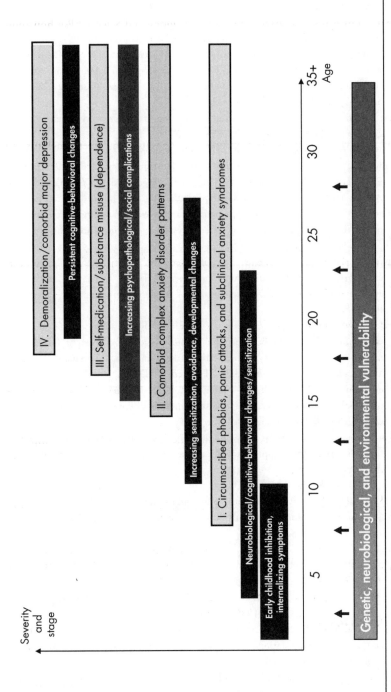

**FIGURE 6–3.** Possible developmental stages (I–IV) and pathways and putative mechanisms.

American Psychiatric Association. Diagnostic and Statistical Manual of Mental Disorders, 3rd Edition, Revised. Washington, DC: American Psychiatric Association, 1987.

American Psychiatric Association. Diagnostic and Statistical Manual of Mental Disorders, 4th Edition. Washington, DC: American Psychiatric Association, 1994.

American Psychiatric Association. Diagnostic and Statistical Manual of Mental Disorders, 4th Edition, Text Revision. Washington, DC: American Psychiatric Association, 2000.

Amir N, Foa EB, Coles ME. Factor structure of the Yale–Brown Obsessive Compulsive Scale. Psychol Assess 1997; 9: 312–316.

Angst J, Merikangas K, Prisig M. Subthreshold syndromes of depression and anxiety in the community. J Clin Psychiatry 1997; 58: 6–10.

Barlow DH. Anxiety and Its Disorders. New York: Guilford, 1988.

Barlow DH. The nature of anxiety: anxiety, depression, and emotional disorders. In Rapee RM, Barlow DH (eds) Chronic Anxiety: Generalized Anxiety Disorder and Mixed Anxiety-Depression. New York: Guilford, 1991, pp. 1–28.

Barlow DH. The nature of anxious apprehension. In Barlow DH (ed) Anxiety and Its Disorders: The Nature and Treatment of Anxiety and Panic. New York: Guilford, 2002, pp. 64–104.

Barlow DH, Di Nardo PA. The diagnosis of generalized anxiety disorder: development, current status, and future directions. In Rapee RM, Barlow DH (eds) Chronic Anxiety: Generalized Anxiety Disorder and Mixed Anxiety-Depression. New York: Guilford, 1991, pp. 95–118.

Beesdo K. Wie entstehen generalisierte ängste? Eine prospektiv-longitudinale, klinisch-epidemiologische Studie bei Jugendlichen und jungen Erwachsenen (The development of generalized anxiety. A prospective-longitudinal, clinical-epidemiologic study among adolescents and young adults). Dresden: TUDpress, 2006.

Bittner A, Goodwin RD, Wittchen H-U, Beesdo K, Höfler M, Lieb R. What characteristics of primary anxiety disorders predict subsequent major depressive disorder? J Clin Psychiatry 2004; 65: 618–626.

Cassano GB, Michelini S, Shear MK, Coli E, Maser JD, Frank E. The panic-agoraphobic spectrum: a descriptive approach to the assessment and treatment of subtle symptoms. Am J Psychiatry 1997; 154: 27–38.

Cassano G, Banti S, Mauri M, Dell'Osso L, Miniati M, Maser J, Shear M, Frank E, Grochocinski V, Rucci P. Internal consistency and discriminant validity of the Structured Clinical Interview for Panic-Agoraphobic Spectrum (SCI-PAS). Int J Methods Psychiatr Res 1999; 8: 138–145.

Chambless DL, Caputo GC, Bright P, Gallagher R. Assessment of fear of fear in agoraphobics: the Body Sensation Questionnaire and the Agoraphobic Cognitions Questionnaire. J Consult Clin Psychol 1984; 52: 1090–1097.

Chambless D, Caputo G, Hasin F, Gracley E, Williams C. The Mobility Inventory for Agoraphobia. Behav Res Ther 1985; 23: 35–44.

Clark DA, Steer RA, Beck AT. Common and specific dimensions of self-reported anxiety and depression: implications for the cognitive and tripartite models. J Abnorm Psychol 1994; 103: 645–654.

Clark LA, Watson D. Tripartite model of anxiety and depression: psychometric evidence and taxonomic implications. J Abnorm Psychol 1991; 100: 316–336.

Clark LA, Watson D, Mineka S. Temperament, personality, and the mood and anxiety disorders. J Abnorm Psychol 1994; 103: 103–116.

Craske MG. Anxiety Disorders: Psychological Approaches to Theory and Treatment. Boulder, CO: Westview Press, 1999.

Craske MG. Origins of Phobias and Anxiety Disorders: Why More Women Than Men? Amsterdam: Elsevier, 2003.

Eifert G, Forsyth J. Acceptance & Commitment Therapy for Anxiety Disorders: A Practitioner's Guide to Using Mindfulness, Acceptance, and Values-Based Behavior Change Strategies. Oakland, CA: New Harbinger Publications, 2005.

Emmelkamp PMG, Wittchen H-U. Specific phobias. In Stress and Fear Circuitry Disorders: Refining the Research Agenda for DSM-V. Andrews G, Charney D, Sirovatka PJ, Regier DA (eds) Arlington, VA: American Psychiatric Association, in press.

Fanselow MS, Lester LS. A functional behavioristic approach to aversively motivated behavior: predatory imminence as a determinant of the topography of defensive behavior. In Bolles RC, Beecher MD (eds) Evolution and Learning. Hillsdale, NJ: Lawrence Erlbaum Associates, 1988, pp. 185–212.

Fava M, Rush A, Alpert J, Carmin C, Balasubramani G, Wisniewski S, Trivedi M, Biggs M, Shores-Wilson K. What clinical and symptom features and comorbid disorders characterize outpatients with anxious major depressive disorder: a replication and extension. Can J Psychiatry 2006; 51: 823–835.

Fergusson D, Horwood L, Boden J. Structure of internalising symptoms in early adulthood. Br J Psychiatry 2006; 489: 540–546.

First MB, Gibbon M. The Structured Clinical Interview for DSM-IV Axis I Disorders (SCID-I) and the Structured Clinical Interview for DSM-IV Axis II Disorders (SCID-II). In Hilsenroth MJ, Segal DL (eds) Comprehensive Handbook of Psychological Assessment, Vol 2: Personality Assessment. Chichester: Wiley, 2004, p. 134.

Frank E, Cassano G, Shear M, Rotondo A, Dell'Osso L, Mauri M, Maser J, Grochocinski V. The spectrum model: a more coherent approach to the complexity of psychiatric symptomatology. CNS Spectr 1998; 3: 23–34.

Frank E, Cyranowski JM, Rucci P, Shear MK, Fagiolini A, Thase ME, Cassano GB, Grochocinski VJ, Kostelnik B, Kupfer DJ. Clinical significance of lifetime panic spectrum symptoms in the treatment of patients with bipolar I disorder. Arch Gen Psychiatry 2002a; 59: 905–911.

Frank E, Shear MK, Rucci P, Cyranowski JM, Endicott J, Fagiolini A, Grochocinski VJ, Houck P, Kupfer DJ, Maser JD, Cassano GB. Influence of panic-agoraphobic spectrum symptoms on treatment response in patients with recurrent major depression. Am J Psychiatry 2002b; 157: 1101–1107.

Frank E, Shear MK, Rucci P, Banti S, Mauri M, Maser JD, Kupfer DJ, Miniati M, Fagiolini A, Cassano GB. Cross-cultural validity of the Structured Clinical Interview for Panic-Agoraphobic Spectrum. Soc Psychiatry Psychiatr Epidemiol 2005; 40: 283–290.

Goldberg D. A dimensional model for common mental disorders. Br J Psychiatry 1996; 168: 44–49.

Goodman WK, Price LH, Rasmussen SA, Mazure C, Fleischmann RL, Hill CL, Heninger GR, Charney DS. The Yale–Brown Obsessive Compulsive Scale. I. Development, use, and reliability. Arch Gen Psychiatry 1989; 46: 1006–1011.

Goodwin RD, Hamilton SP. Panic attack as a marker of core psychopathological processes. Psychopathology 2001; 24: 278–288.

Goodwin RD, Roy-Byrne P. Panic and suicidal ideation and suicide attempts: results from the National Comorbidity Survey. Depress Anxiety 2006; 23: 124–132.

Goodwin RD, Lieb R, Höfler M, Pfister H, Bittner A, Beesdo K, Wittchen H-U. Panic attack as a risk factor for severe psychopathology. Am J Psychiatry 2004; 161: 2207–2214.

Grant BF, Hasin DS, Stinson FS, Dawson DA, Ruan WJ, Goldstein RB, Smith SM, Saha TS, Huang B. Prevalence, correlates, co-morbidity, and comparative disability of DSM-IV generalized anxiety disorder in the USA: results from the National Epidemiologic Survey on Alcohol and Related Conditions. Psychol Med 2005; 35: 1747–1759.

Gregory AM, Caspi A, Moffitt TE, Koenen K, Eley TC, Poulton R. Juvenile mental health histories of adults with anxiety disorders. Am J Psychiatry 2007; 164: 301–308.

Haffner S. Diabetes and the metabolic syndrome—when is it best to intervene to prevent? Atheroscler Suppl 2006; 7: 3–10.

Hamilton M. The assessment of anxiety-states by rating. Br J Med Psychol 1959; 32: 50–55.

Hollander E. Obsessive-compulsive disorder and spectrum across the life span. International Journal of Psychiatry in Clinical Practice 2005; 9: 79–86.

Kessler RC, Brandenburg N, Lane M, Roy-Byrne P, Stang PE, Stein DJ, Wittchen H-U. Rethinking the duration requirement for generalized anxiety disorder: evidence from the National Comorbidity Survey Replication. Psychol Med 2005; 35: 1–10.

Klein DF. Anxiety reconceptualized. In Klein DF, Rabkin JG (eds) Anxiety: New Research and Changing Concepts. New York: Raven, 1981, pp. 235–263.

Knäuper B. Age differences in question and response order effects. In Schwarz N, Park DC, Knäuper B, Sudman S (eds) Cognition, Aging, and Self-Reports. Hove: Psychology Press/Erlbaum (UK) Taylor & Francis, 1999, pp. 341–363.

Krueger RF. Structure of common mental disorders. Arch Gen Psychiatry 1999; 56: 921–926.

Krueger RF, Caspi A, Moffitt TE, Silva PA. The structure and stability of common mental disorders (DSM-III-R): a longitudinal-epidemiological study. J Abnorm Psychol 1998; 107: 216–227.

Lara DR, Pinto O, Akiskal KK, Akiskal HS. Toward an integrative model of the spectrum of mood, behavioral and personality disorders based on fear and anger traits: I. Clinical implications. J Affect Disord 2006; 94: 67–87.

Liebowitz MR. Social phobia. Modern Problems of Pharmacopsychiatry 1987; 22: 141–173.

Manfredini D, Landi N, Fantoni F, Segu M, Bosco M. Anxiety symptoms in clinically diagnosed bruxers. J Oral Rehabil 2005; 32: 584–588.

Martini C, Trincavelli M, Tuscano D, Carmassi C, Ciapparelli A, Lucacchini A, Cassano G, Dell'Osso L. Serotonin-mediated phosphorylation of extracellular regulated kinases in platelets of patients with panic disorder versus controls. Neurochem Int 2004; 44: 627–639.

Mundt JC, Marks IM, Shear MK, Greist JM. The Work and Social Adjustment Scale: a simple measure of impairment in functioning. Br J Psychiatry 2002; 180: 461–464.

Overall J, Gorman D. The Brief Psychiatric Rating Scale. Psychol Rep 1962; 10: 799–812.

Reed V, Wittchen H-U. DSM-IV panic attacks and panic disorder in a community sample of adolescents and young adults: how specific are panic attacks? J Psychiatr Res 1998; 32: 335–345.

Reiss S, Peterson RA, Gursky DM, McNally RJ. Anxiety sensitivity, anxiety frequency, and the prediction of fearfulness. Behav Res Ther 1986; 24: 1–8.

Ruscio AM, Lane M, Roy-Byrne P, Stang PE, Stein DJ, Wittchen H-U, Kessler RC. Should excessive worry be required for a diagnosis of generalized anxiety disorder? results from the US National Comorbidity Survey Replication. Psychol Med 2005; 35: 1761–1772.

Ruscio AM, Chiu WT, Roy-Byrne P, Stang PE, Stein DJ, Wittchen H-U, Kessler RC. Broadening the definition of generalized anxiety disorder: effects on prevalence and associations with other disorders in the National Comorbidity Survey Replication. J Anxiety Disord 2007; 21: 667–676.

Shear K, Frank E, Rucci P, Fagiolini DA, Grochocinski VJ, Houck P, Cassano GB, Kupfer DJ, Endicott J, Maser JD, Mauri M, Banti S. Panic-agoraphobic spectrum: reliability and validity of assessment instruments. J Psychiatr Res 2001a; 35: 59–66.

Shear K, Rucci P, Williams J, Frank E, Grochocinski V, Vander Bilt J, Houck P, Wang T. Reliability and validity of the Panic Disorder Severity Scale: replication and extension. J Psychiatr Res 2001b; 35: 293–296.

Shear K, Belnap BH, Mazumdar S, Houck P, Rollman BL. Generalized Anxiety Disorder Severity Scale (GADSS): a preliminary validation study. Depress Anxiety 2006; 23: 77–82.

Sheehan D. Sheehan Disability Scale (1983). In Rush A Jr, Pincus H, First M, Blacker D, Endicott J, Keith S, Phillips K, Ryan N, Smith G Jr, Tsuang M, Widiger T, Zarin D (eds) Task Force for the Handbook of Psychiatric Measures. Washington, DC: American Psychiatric Press, 2000, p. 113, test on CD; Chapter 8: Mental health status, functioning, and disabilities measures.

Spielberger CD, Gorusch RL, Lushene RH. State-Trait Anxiety Inventory. Palo Alto: Consulting Psychologists Press, 1970.

Spitzer RL, Williams JBW, Gibbon M, First MB. The Structured Clinical Interview for DSM-III-R (SCID). 1. History, rationale, and description. Arch Gen Psychiatry 1992; 49: 624–629.

Taylor S, Cox BJ. An expanded Anxiety Sensitivity Index: evidence for a hierarchic structure in a clinical sample. J Anxiety Disord 1998; 12: 463–483.

Trivedi MH, Rush AJ, Wisniewski SR, Nierenberg AA, Warden D, Ritz L, Norquist G, Howland RH, Lebowitz B, McGrath PJ, Shores-Wilson K, Biggs MM, Balasubramani GK, Fava M, Team SDS. Evaluation of outcomes with citalopram for depression using measurement-based care in STAR*D: implications for clinical practice. Am J Psychiatry 2006; 163: 28–40.

Vollebergh WAM, Iedema J, Bijl RV, de Graaf R, Smit F, Ormel J. The structure and stability of common mental disorders. The NEMESIS Study. Arch Gen Psychiatry 2001; 58: 597–603.

Watson D. Rethinking the mood and anxiety disorders: a quantitative hierarchical model for DSM-V. J Abnorm Psychol 2005; 114: 522–536.

Watson D, Friend R. Measurement of social-evaluative anxiety. J Consult Clin Psychol 1969; 33: 448–457.

Watson D, Weber K, Smith Assenheimer J, Clark LA, Strauss ME, McCormick R. Testing a tripartite model: I. Evaluating the convergent and discriminant validity of anxiety and depression symptom scales. J Abnorm Psychol 1995; 104: 3–14.

Widiger TA. A dimensional model of psychopathology. Psychopathology 2005; 38: 211–214.

Widiger TA, Clark LA. Toward DSM-V and the classification of psychopathology. Psychol Bull 2000; 126: 946–963.

Widiger TA, Samuel DB. Diagnostic categories or dimensions? a question for the Diagnostic and Statistical Manual of Mental Disorders, Fifth Edition. J Abnorm Psychol 2005; 114: 494–504.

Wiersma D, de Jong A, Ormel J. The Groningen Social Disabilities Schedule: development, relationship with the ICIDH and psychometric properties. Int J Rehabil Res 1988; 11: 213–224.

Wiersma D, de Jong A, Kraaijkamp HJM. GSDS-II. The Groningen Social Disabilities Schedule, second version. Manual, questionnaire and rating form. Groningen: Department of Social Psychiatry, University of Groningen, 1990.

Wittchen H-U, Höfler M, Merikangas KR. Towards the identification of core psychopathological processes? Arch Gen Psychiatry 1999; 56: 929–931.

Wittchen H-U, Lecrubier Y, Beesdo K, Nocon A. Relationships among anxiety disorders: patterns and implications. In Nutt DJ, Ballenger JC (eds) Anxiety Disorders. Oxford: Blackwell Science, 2003, pp. 25–37.

World Health Organization (WHO). Composite International Diagnostic Interview (CIDI). Geneva: WHO, 1990.

World Health Organization (WHO). World Health Organization Disability Assessment Schedule (WHODAS II). Geneva: WHO, 2000.

Zigmond A, Snaith R. The hospital anxiety and depression scale. Acta Psychiatr Scand 1983; 67: 361–370.

Zinbarg RE, Barlow DH. Structure of anxiety and the anxiety disorders: a hierarchical model. J Abnorm Psychol 1996; 105: 181–193.

# 7

# SYNTHESIZING DIMENSIONAL AND CATEGORICAL APPROACHES TO PERSONALITY DISORDERS

## Refining the Research Agenda for DSM-V Axis II

Robert F. Krueger, Ph.D.
Andrew E. Skodol, M.D.
W. John Livesley, M.D., Ph.D.
Patrick E. Shrout, Ph.D.
Yueqin Huang, M.D., M.P.H., Ph.D.

The personality disorders (PDs) field has taken a leading role in contemplating the utility of dimensional approaches to the diagnosis of mental disorders (Krueger et al. 2005; Kupfer et al. 2002). A previous American Psychiatric Institute for Research and Education (APIRE) meeting focused specifically on dimensional approaches to PDs (Widiger et al. 2005), and many advantages of dimensional

Reprinted with permission from Krueger R, Skodol AE, Livesley WJ, Shrout PE, Huang Y. "Synthesizing Dimensional and Categorical Approaches to Personality Disorders: Refining the Research Agenda for DSM-V Axis II." *International Journal of Methods in Psychiatric Research* 2007; 16(S1): S65–S73.

approaches to PDs are well documented in the literature. For example, dimensional representations of specific DSM-IV (American Psychiatric Association 1994) PDs and other dimensional representations of personality pathology are better predictors of functional impairment when compared with categorical representations of DSM-IV PDs in treatment-seeking patients (Morey et al., in press; Skodol et al. 2005).

Depending on the exact details, however, a novel dimensional system for PDs in DSM-V could represent an unnecessarily abrupt departure from the constructs described in DSM-IV, some of which have garnered extensive clinical and research interest. Although implementation of dimensions in DSM-V is called for by the research literature, this implementation will likely be more successful if it is an orderly and logical progression from DSM-IV (cf. Helzer et al. 2006).

With this backdrop in mind, we set out to sketch an approach that might be considered a starting point for discussion related to Axis II of DSM-V. Our intent is not to advocate for a specific proposal, as such advocacy would be premature at this early stage in the development of DSM-V. Rather, our intent is to provide some examples that emerged from our discussion that we hope will be useful in catalyzing deliberations and framing initial field testing.

A central theme that emerged in our work was the importance of synthesizing various approaches in the literature, in particular, categorical and dimensional approaches to PDs. We begin by describing the foundation of the approach we developed in our discussion: a set of core elements for the description of the diversity of personalities seen in clinical settings.

# Core Elements for Personality Description in DSM

The current DSM-IV system for PDs entails 10 categorical disorders. Embedded in these 10 disorders are 79 descriptive criteria (not counting ancillary criteria such as exclusionary criteria). A thorough differential diagnosis of the 10 DSM-IV PDs would involve considering the applicability of each of these 79 criteria to a specific patient. Although clinicians may not typically evaluate all 79 criteria, maintaining high fidelity to DSM per se would involve taking on this rather significant burden. For example, when the DSM PD criteria are operationalized in comprehensive semistructured interviews, such interviews need to cover each PD criterion to maintain fidelity to the DSM system (Widiger et al. 2006). Indeed, front-line clinicians often simplify the diagnostic task by matching their perceptions of patients with conceptual prototypes (Shedler and Westen 2004), as opposed to evaluating numerous criteria individually. One of the reasons for taking this shortcut may be the burden created by the 79 distinct criteria on the current Axis II. Moreover, in spite of the large number of criteria on DSM-IV Axis II, there is evidence that the

10 disorders delineated by these criteria do not exhaust the diversity of personality pathology seen in clinical practice (Westen and Arkowitz-Westen 1998). This may be one reason why PD not otherwise specified is a prevalent diagnosis (Verheul and Widiger 2004).

Fortunately, research on the fine-grained structure of personality pathology points to a smaller number of fundamental elements or "facets" that can be used to provide a comprehensive description of abnormal personality. Although a number of systems have been described in the literature, they are notably congruent, especially in the way they delineate broad domains of personality functioning (Markon et al. 2005; Widiger and Simonsen 2005). As an example, we focus here on one specific set of facets, those delineated by the Dimensional Assessment of Personality Pathology (DAPP; Livesley, submitted for publication).

The DAPP system consists of 30 facet-level constructs. These constructs were generated by starting with trait descriptions and behavioral acts that were characteristic of PDs as described in DSM-III and in the broader literature on personality pathology (Livesley, submitted for publication). A series of psychometric and behavior genetic analyses (described in greater detail by Livesley, submitted for publication) were used to refine the initial set of descriptions, and this process resulted in the specific facets of the current DAPP system. Table 7–1 presents names of the facets and brief vignettes summarizing the characteristics of persons who have the personality features captured by the facets. In addition, the facets in Table 7–1 are arranged into four broad groups derived from research on the empirical structure of the facets (Livesley et al. 1998): emotional dysregulation, dissocial behavior, inhibitedness, and compulsivity.

The personality features described in Table 7–1 provide a starting point for translating facets into descriptive elements for DSM-V per se (Livesley, submitted for publication). Specifically, DSM-V could include descriptions of each facet, akin to those in Table 7–1. In addition, DSM-V would provide guidance to the user regarding how to rate the facets in describing a specific patient or research participant. Although a number of approaches could be considered, a straightforward option is portrayed in Table 7–2, involving a four-point scale with scale points linked to how characteristic the facet is of the person in general. An even simpler option is to rate each facet as present versus absent, but the disadvantage of this approach is that more information is contained in the more fine-grained four-point scale portrayed in Table 7–2.

Although we have focused here on the DAPP system for delineating the facet-level structure of personality pathology, it is important to note that we could have used a number of other prominent systems as examples (see Widiger and Simonsen 2005, for a review). Indeed, these various systems are well integrated in a hierarchical fashion, with different systems emphasizing different levels of breadth versus specificity in the description of abnormal personality features (Markon et al. 2005). The use of any level of this hierarchy as an example would serve to make the general point

**TABLE 7–1.** The 30 facets of the DAPP Model

| Secondary domain | Primary facet trait | Defining features |
|---|---|---|
| Emotional dysregulation | Anxiousness | Trait anxiety; rumination; indecisiveness; guilt proneness |
| | Emotional reactivity | Emotional lability; irritability; labile anger |
| | Emotional intensity | Expresses feelings intensely; experiences strong feelings; overreacts emotionally; exaggerates emotional significance of events |
| | Pessimistic anhedonia | Anhedonia; pervasive pessimism; feelings of emptiness and boredom |
| | Submissiveness | Submissive; needs advice and reassurance about all courses of action; suggestible |
| | Insecure attachment | Fears losing attachments; coping depends on presence of attachment figure; urgently seeks proximity with attachment figure when stressed; strongly protests separations; intolerant of aloneness |
| | Social apprehensiveness | Fears hurt and rejection; poor social skills; desires affiliative relationships |
| | Need for approval | Strong need for demonstrations of acceptance and approval; constantly seeks reassurance that he/she is a worthy person |
| | Cognitive dysregulation | Depersonalization or derealization; schizotypal cognition; brief stress psychosis |
| | Oppositional | Oppositional behaviors |
| | Self-harming acts | Deliberate self-damaging acts, e.g., self-mutilation, drug overdoses |
| | Self-harming ideas | Frequent thoughts about hurting self and suicide |

**TABLE 7–1.**   The 30 facets of the DAPP Model *(continued)*

| Secondary domain | Primary facet trait | Defining features |
| --- | --- | --- |
| Dissocial behavior | Narcissism | Grandiose; seeks attention; needs to be admired |
| | Exploitativeness | Takes advantage of others for personal gain; charming and ingratiating when suits own purpose; believes that others are easily manipulated or conned; considers self to be adroit at taking advantage of others |
| | Sadism | Sadistic; contemptuous |
| | Conduct problems | Violence; addictive behavior; juvenile antisocial behavior; failure to adopt social norms |
| | Hostile-dominance | Interpersonally hostile; dominant |
| | Sensation seeking | Sensation seeking; reckless |
| | Impulsivity | Does things on the spur of the moment; many actions unplanned or without a lot of thought about the consequence; fails to follow established plans; appears not to learn from experience (impulsivity overrules previous experiences) |
| | Suspiciousness | Suspicious; hypervigilant |
| | Egocentrism | Preoccupied with self; perceptions dominated by own point of view, interests, and concerns; defines and pursues own needs without regard for those of others; believes he/she knows what is best for others |

**TABLE 7–1.**  The 30 facets of the DAPP Model *(continued)*

| Secondary domain | Primary facet trait | Defining features |
|---|---|---|
| Inhibitedness | Low affiliation | Seeks out situations that do not include other people; declines opportunities to socialize; has few friends; does not initiate social contact |
|  | Avoidant attachment | Avoids attachment relationships; fearful of attachments; does not seek out others when stressed or distressed; shows little reaction to separations or reunions |
|  | Attachment need | Desires attachment relationships; distressed by lack of intimacy |
|  | Inhibited sexuality | Lacks interest in sexuality; derives little pleasure from sexual experiences; fearful of sexual expression |
|  | Self-containment | Reluctant to self-disclose; self-reliant and self-sufficient |
|  | Inhibited emotional expression | Does not display feelings; avoids emotionally arousing situations; does not reveal angry or positive feelings; appears unemotional |
|  | Lack of empathy | Lacks empathy; remorseless; lack of responsibility |
| Compulsivity | Orderliness | Orderly; precise |
|  | Conscientiousness | Strong sense of duty and obligation; completes all tasks thoroughly and meticulously |

---

**TABLE 7–2.**   An example scale for applying facet descriptors to specific persons

Specify how applicable the facet is to the person:

(1)  Highly uncharacteristic: the facet describes thoughts, feelings, and behaviors that are rarely if ever seen in the person

(2)  Somewhat uncharacteristic: the facet describes the thoughts, feelings, and behaviors of the person on a few occasions, but less than half of the time the person was observed

(3)  Somewhat characteristic: the facet describes the thoughts, feelings, and behaviors of the person more than half of the time the person was observed

(4)  Highly characteristic: the facet exemplifies the typical thoughts, feelings, and behaviors of the person and is a pervasive part of the person's personality

---

that a comprehensive set of facet-level personality pathology descriptors is a tractable goal for DSM-V. Indeed, if the DSM-V PD workgroup decides to pursue the ideas we have described here, a key task will be to carefully examine facet-level constructs associated with various systems to arrive at the most clinically optimal set of facets. Widiger and Simonsen (2005) came to a similar conclusion, and they have detailed a number of considerations that are relevant to this task (e.g., overlap among facet scales and clinical relevance). In addition, the systems reviewed by Widiger and Simonsen (2005) are diverse in their goals and origins (e.g., describing "normal" personality traits versus being designed specifically to describe both "normal" and "abnormal" personality traits), and these differences between the systems are also important to consider in arriving at a clinically optimal set of facets. For example, the prototype matching system developed by Westen et al. (2006b) provides an explicit means of linking clinically rich facet-level descriptions with the need to classify specific patients via their match to diagnostic prototypes.

There are a number of advantages of a smaller number of core descriptive facets for DSM-V over the 79 criteria of DSM-IV. One notable advantage is that these facets simplify the task of PD assessment in both research and in the clinic. Rather than having to consider 79 criteria, the clinician or researcher interested in comprehensive PD assessment only needs to consider 30 facets. In addition, a comprehensive set of facets provides a comprehensive set of targets to further empirical research on PD. Indeed, a number of key investigations could be pursued as part of a PD field trial to help refine the facets prior to finalizing them for DSM-V. For example, the facets described in Table 7–1 are intended to be rated by an observer (e.g., a clinician) but were developed initially through self-report. Correspondence between raters is not perfect and the discrepancies between raters may be of clinical importance (see Oltmanns and Turkheimer 2006 for a review of relevant research in the PD domain). Field trial studies could therefore be pursued to understand how to best combine data on the facets from multiple raters. Similarly, the facets may function differently in different cultural groups, or across genders, in terms of how they reflect underlying domains of personality functioning. Sensitivity to such group differences is a core concern in work leading up to DSM-V (Alarcon et al. 2002), and a set of preliminary facets provides comprehensive targets for studying the ways in which culture influences the expression of personality pathology.

A comprehensive set of PD facets for DSM-V also provides a means of implementing an important aspect of DSM-IV that we see as underutilized. Specifically, DSM-IV notes that maladaptive personality traits that do not constitute a formal PD can be listed on Axis II, but DSM-IV does not provide an empirically derived set of traits to use for this purpose. Because personality and psychopathology are intimately intertwined (see, e.g., Krueger and Tackett 2006), a formal system for describing the personality of any patient, independent of the extent to which that person could be said to have a PD, is likely to be quite helpful. For example, Harkness and McNulty (2002) described a number of ways in which personality trait concepts can be useful in clinical work, beyond their utility in conceptualizing PDs, including selecting intervention approaches that match the patient's personality. Consider two cases of "garden-variety unipolar depression" that differ on the facet of oppositionality. The more oppositional unipolar depressive patient would be less likely to comply naturally with the extra-session demands of a cognitive-behavioral approach, and the treatment plan for this patient could be adjusted to take into account issues with compliance—issues that are less likely to affect intervention with the less oppositional patient.

Another important aspect of a comprehensive set of PD facets is the ability to translate back to key PDs described in DSM-IV. The facets can be combined to form PD prototypes, akin to the way the 79 criteria of DSM-IV are combined to form the 10 DSM-IV PD categories.

# Combining Facets to Describe Personality Disorder Prototypes

The PD categories of DSMs since DSM-III (American Psychiatric Association 1980) have been criticized on various grounds, but it is nevertheless the case that some of these categories describe clinical personality constructs in which there is substantial interest. Blashfield and Intoccia (2000) conducted a very informative systematic review of articles listed on MEDLINE to determine if specific DSM-defined PDs were linked to a growing as opposed to a stagnant or shrinking literature. They found that most DSM-defined PDs were associated with very little literature. Only three PDs (schizotypal, borderline, and antisocial) were associated with literatures that were "alive and well" and only borderline was associated with a literature that was not only alive, but also growing.

**TABLE 7–3.** Prototypical borderline personality features

| | |
|---|---|
| Anxiousness | Impulsivity |
| Emotional reactivity | Insecure attachment |
| Emotional intensity | Pessimistic anhedonia |
| Attachment need | Self-harming acts |
| Cognitive dysregulation | Self-harming ideas |

This variation in the level of interest in specific DSM-IV PDs needs to be taken into account in working toward DSM-V. In particular, there are likely to be understandable objections to a DSM-V PD section that lacks criteria for PDs that have generated substantial interest and research. Fortunately, a comprehensive set of personality facets provides a way of linking the burgeoning literature on dimensional representations of PDs with literatures on specific categorical PD constructs. In particular, facets such as those portrayed in Table 7–1 can be combined to describe the configurations of personality features that exemplify prototypical cases of specific PDs. We will focus here on borderline PD as an example because, as noted by Blashfield and Intoccia (2000), this is the single example of a DSM-defined PD in which interest seems to be growing. Clearly, the DSM-V PD workgroup will also have to think very carefully about this issue with reference to other PDs delineated in DSM-IV and in the broader clinical literature.

Table 7–3 shows the authors' judgment of the DAPP facets that, when combined, define the prototypical borderline PD case (see also Pukrop 2002 for a study of the DAPP in borderline PD patients). These facets could be listed in DSM-V as diagnostic criteria for borderline PD in the same way that the nine criteria for borderline PD are listed in DSM-IV. By adding up scores on these facets, the user of DSM-V would generate a dimensional score representing the extent to which a given patient resembles the personality of the prototypical borderline PD patient (cf. Oldham and Skodol 2000; Westen et al. 2006b). However, this score would not be the equivalent of a borderline PD diagnosis. Rather, we see the concept of a diagnosable PD as involving the combination of personality traits and a separate but complementary evaluation of personality dysfunction.

# General Personality Disorder Criteria for DSM-V

One of the deeper and more challenging issues in psychopathology research relates to demarcating the distinction between normality and abnormality. This problem is especially acute for PDs by the very nature of the concept. The term "personality disorder" suggests that something everyone has (a personality) has gone awry (become disordered); the term itself highlights the importance of conceptualizing the distinction between individual differences (personality traits) and the ways in which personality mechanisms in a specific individual fail to perform their intended functions (personality disorders). One way of dealing with this problem is to simply define PD as extreme personality traits in the statistical sense. This solution is generally considered inadequate because it leaves the question of what constitutes "extremity." Widiger et al. (2002) discuss how extremity could be defined as the point along a personality continuum where associated impairment becomes clinically significant. What it means for something to become "clinically significant" can be informed by data on the correlates and consequences of personality traits, such that this approach neatly combines evidence about personality variation with evidence about clinical correlates of personality traits. This is an appealing model, and it has been successful in application to other clinical phenomena (e.g., defining the level of IQ that constitutes cognitive impairment; defining the level of blood pressure that constitutes hypertension).

However, it is also useful to consider how PD may constitute something more than clinically significant extremity of personality (Livesley and Jang 2005). In particular, the notion of disorder implies a mechanism that is not functioning in the manner intended—a mechanism that is dysfunctional and that is keeping the individual from functioning adaptively (cf. Wakefield 1992). In particular, as discussed by Livesley and Jang (2005), the consequences of personality for adaptive functioning in adulthood need to be considered in defining PD. Personality involves not only traits—nomothetic constructs that differentiate people—but also intrapsychic systems designed to pursue valued and need-fulfilling life tasks (Westen et al. 2006a). Adult life tasks include creating stable and cohesive working models of the self and others that allow a person to be able to get along (e.g., pursue close and meaningful intimate relationships), while still being able to get ahead (e.g., working to establish oneself in a chosen occupation). The inability to pursue these fundamental tasks of adult life is central to clinical observations about the intrapsychic structure of personality in personality-disordered patients, and diminished probability of success in these tasks is associated with personality pathology (Skodol et al. 2005).

This distinction between what a person's personality is in the nomothetic "between-persons" sense (personality traits) and how it can fail to do what it is designed to do in adulthood (a "within-person" PD) is important for DSM-V. Indeed, we would argue that the transition to DSM-V provides an important opportunity to better articulate the concepts of both "personality" and "disorder." As we described earlier, a specific model of facet-level personality traits would provide a notable advance over DSM-IV in the sense that DSM-IV encourages recording of traits but lacks provision of a set of trait concepts for clinical and research use. Along with this, however, we would suggest that DSM-V include a new set of general criteria for PD. Our specific suggested criteria are listed in Table 7–4.

The set listed in Table 7–4 is somewhat simpler than the set listed in DSM-IV, and its adoption would involve deleting criteria A, B, C, D, and E from DSM-IV

---

**TABLE 7–4.** Suggested general diagnostic criteria for a personality disorder (PD) in DSM-V

---

A. Persistent inability to accomplish one or more of the following basic tasks of adult life:

    1) Establishment of coherent and adaptive working models of the self and others (e.g., is capable of formulating a clear and consistent sense of her/ his goals and values in life; perceives other people as coherent entities)

    2) Establishment of intimate relationships and activities (e.g., a longer term relationship that involves mutual emotional support)

    3) Establishment of occupational relationships and activities (e.g., employment that provides a stable source of income)

B. 18 years of age or older

C. The inability to accomplish life tasks is not due to the direct physiological effects of a substance (e.g., a drug of abuse, a medication) or a general medical condition (e.g., head trauma)

D. Specify features of the PD by recording facet traits rated as highly characteristic or highly uncharacteristic.

E. Specify the degree of correspondence of the PD to personality prototypes by recording the number of prototypical features present (rated as highly characteristic or highly uncharacteristic). If more than a critical number of features (determined by a field trial) of a personality prototype are present, record the prototype as the subtype of personality disorder.

---

(criterion F from DSM-IV is represented in Table 7–4 as criterion C). DSM-IV criterion A is eliminated because it relates to personality per se (referring, e.g., to persistent deviant behavior, such as deficient impulse control). We have eliminated this criterion because it refers to nomothetic personality variation, which would be encoded by facet traits, such as those in Table 7–1, as opposed to disorder per se. DSM-IV criterion B requires that the personality style referred to by criterion A be pervasive, and this idea of personality consistency is covered in Table 7–4 by criterion D, requiring at least one facet trait that is rated highly characteristic or highly uncharacteristic. DSM-IV criterion C describes clinically significant distress or impairment, and this idea of impairment is covered in Table 7–4 by criterion A, which reflects impaired ability to accomplish basic life tasks, a clinically significant problem. DSM-IV criterion D requires the PD to be stable and of long duration and to be traceable back to adolescence or early adulthood. We eliminated this criterion because the stability of personality features is contained in Table 7–4, criterion D, via the facet rating scale.

    DSM-IV criterion E requires the PD to not be a "manifestation or consequence" of another mental disorder. We eliminated this criterion because it is unclear how to establish that one mental disorder is a "manifestation or consequence" of another mental disorder (see Boyd et al. 1984 for a classic discussion of the practical difficulties inherent in implementing such exclusionary criteria). For example: Must one disorder (B) always occur after another (A) to be considered a consequence? This sort of mechanistic co-occurrence is not typically observed in data on mental disorders, so then does "consequence status" require some probabilistic relationship between A and B over time? What probability of B after A is sufficient to consider B to be a "consequence" of A, and what temporal sequence is required? Such exclusionary criteria were attempted in DSM-III and mostly eliminated in subsequent DSMs because it is essentially impossible to operationalize such criteria meaningfully. At the very least, this criterion (E) is subject to multiple interpretations, and such ambiguity is not helpful in creating reliable criteria for psychopathology.

In addition to elimination of criteria from DSM-IV, Table 7–4 suggests the inclusion of new criteria for DSM-V. Criterion A operationalizes the ideas we described earlier about how PD involves inability to accomplish basic tasks of adult life. Writing a concise description of criterion A(1) of the sort that is in Table 7–4 was especially challenging because the result is somewhat telegraphic relative to the richness of the concept we mean to convey. What it means to "perceive other people in coherent ways" has been the subject of extensive clinical scholarship that is not easily reduced to a straightforward DSM-style criterion (indeed, one could argue that deficits in the ability to conceptualize others' minds and motives coherently form the crux of an entire influential school of thought on clinical psychopathology, object relations [Greenberg and Mitchell 1983]). This problem could be dealt with in DSM-V by including accompanying text that describes in as clear and coherent a way as possible the specific and objective clinical evidence that corresponds to criterion A(1). Some may object that a criterion like A(1) backslides into the vagueness that plagued DSM prior to DSM-III, but we feel A(1) is too central to the clinical nature of personality pathology to not struggle with its inclusion.

Criterion B requires that the individual receiving a PD diagnosis be at least 18 years of age. In DSM-IV, a diagnosis of PD is allowed in individuals under 18 years of age, but this situation is deemed "relatively unusual," the PD features need to be present for at least a year, and such features are described as rarely persisting into adult life. This discomfort with assigning a PD diagnosis to minors is understandable, and by our definition, the concept of PD does not apply to minors because they have not yet faced the basic tasks of adult life. Nevertheless, characterizing the personalities of children and adolescents is important in both clinical and research settings, in part because personality is systematically related to psychopathology in individuals younger than 18 (Shiner 2005; Tackett and Krueger 2005). Our proposal provides a means to facilitate clinical and research use of personality concepts through the facet traits and personality prototypes, which can be used regardless of the presence versus absence of a diagnosable adult PD.

Criterion C in Table 7–4 is criterion F of DSM-IV, as noted earlier. This criterion is preserved because it is obviously clinically important to distinguish personality pathology from the direct effects of CNS trauma. Criterion D in Table 7–4 requires that the user of DSM record the personality features of the specific PD. Criterion D also requires the PD to involve at least one personality feature that is sufficiently florid to receive a rating of highly characteristic or uncharacteristic. In addition, criterion E requires that the user of DSM specify correspondence with any personality prototypes that might be developed for DSM-V, akin to the borderline prototype described in Table 7–3. By recording the number of prototypical features present, DSM would include a dimensional representation of prototype resemblance (cf. Oldham and Skodol 2000). Criterion E also specifies that the user assign a subtype label to the PD if a yet-to-be-determined number of all of the features that comprise a prototype are present. Thresholds for subtype status could be set based on data collected as part of a field trial process. For example, the number of prototype criteria present could be used to predict key clinical outcomes (e.g., suicidality) and thresholds set accordingly (cf. Widiger et al. 2002).

According to this system, the PD diagnosis in DSM-V could be moved to Axis I, and Axis II of DSM-V could be revised to correspond to facet traits such as those in Table 7–1, a rating scale such as the one in Table 7–2, and prototypes such as the borderline prototype in Table 7–3 and others that may be developed by the DSM-V PD workgroup. This could be controversial but may also have a number of fundamental benefits. First, a multiaxial diagnosis would routinely involve evaluating the patient's personality features, which would be recorded on Axis II regardless of whether a PD was present. This corresponds well to the original intent in DSM-III of recognizing personality as an aspect of any patient by recording it on an axis separate from the axis used to record current diagnoses. Second, the diagnosis of PD would be given a status equivalent to that of other mental disorders. This could prove fundamentally helpful in facilitating third-party payment for professional services to assist PD patients and in recognizing PDs as debilitating conditions with social costs similar to—if not greater than—those of other major mental disorders (Skodol et al. 2005). It also recognizes calls to conceptualize some features of PD in terms of their link with features of Axis I disorders (e.g., a desire for change and subjective suffering in borderline PD patients; Tyrer 1999). More broadly, moving PD to Axis I would recognize research showing that PDs are more similar to than different from Axis I disorders in many diverse respects (Krueger 2005).

# References

Alarcon RD, Bell CC, Kirmayer LJ, Lin KM, Ustun B, Wisner KL. Beyond the funhouse mirrors: research agenda on culture and psychiatric diagnosis. In Kupfer DJ, First MB, Regier DA (eds) A Research Agenda for DSM-V. Washington, DC: American Psychiatric Association, 2002, pp. 219–281.

American Psychiatric Association. Diagnostic and Statistical Manual of Mental Disorders, 3rd Edition. Washington, DC: American Psychiatric Association, 1980.

American Psychiatric Association. Diagnostic and Statistical Manual of Mental Disorders, 4th Edition. Washington, DC: American Psychiatric Association, 1994.

Blashfield RK, Intoccia V. Growth of the literature on the topic of personality disorders. Am J Psychiatry 2000; 157: 472–473.

Boyd JH, Burke JD, Gruenberg E, Holzer CE, Rae DS, George LK, Karno M, Stoltzman R, McEvoy L, Nestadt G. Exclusion criteria of DSM-III: a study of co-occurrence of hierarchy-free syndromes. Arch Gen Psychiatry 1984; 41: 983–989.

Greenberg JR, Mitchell SA. Object Relations in Psychoanalytic Theory. Cambridge, MA: Harvard University Press, 1983.

Harkness AR, McNulty JL. Implications of individual differences science for clinical work on personality disorders. In Costa PT Jr, Widiger TA (eds) Personality Disorders and the Five-Factor Model of Personality. Washington, DC: American Psychological Association, 2002.

Helzer JE, Kraemer HC, Krueger RF. The feasibility and need for dimensional psychiatric diagnoses. Psychol Med 2006; 36: 1671–1680.

Krueger RF. Continuity of Axes I and II: toward a unified model of personality, personality disorders, and clinical disorders. J Personal Disord 2005; 19: 233–261.

Krueger RF, Tackett JL (eds). Personality and Psychopathology. New York: Guilford, 2006.

Krueger RF, Watson D, Barlow DH. Introduction to the special section: toward a dimensionally based taxonomy of psychopathology. J Abnorm Psychol 2005; 114: 491–493.

Kupfer DJ, First MB, Regier DA (eds). A Research Agenda for DSM-V. Washington, DC: American Psychiatric Association, 2002.

Livesley WJ. A framework for integrating dimensional and categorical classifications of personality disorder (submitted for publication).

Livesley WJ, Jang KL. Differentiating normal, abnormal, and disordered personality. European Journal of Personality 2005; 19: 257–268.

Livesley WJ, Jang KL, Vernon PA. Phenotypic and genetic structure of traits delineating personality disorder. Arch Gen Psychiatry 1998; 55: 941–948.

Markon KE, Krueger RF, Watson D. Delineating the structure of normal and abnormal personality: an integrative hierarchical approach. J Pers Soc Psychol 2005; 88: 139–157.

Morey LC, Hopwood CJ, Gunderson JG, Skodol AE, Shea MT, Yen S, Stout RL, Zanarini MC, Grilo CM, Sanislow CA, McGlashan TH. Comparison of alternative models for personality disorders. Psychol Med (in press).

Oldham JM, Skodol AE. Charting the future of Axis II. J Personal Disord 2000; 14: 17–29.

Oltmanns TF, Turkheimer E. Perceptions of self and others regarding pathological personality traits. In Krueger RF, Tackett JL (eds) Personality and Psychopathology. New York: Guilford, 2006, pp. 71–111.

Pukrop R. Dimensional personality profiles of borderline personality disorder in comparison with other personality disorders and healthy controls. J Personal Disord 2002; 16: 135–147.

Shedler J, Westen D. Refining personality disorder diagnosis: integrating science and practice. Am J Psychiatry 2004; 161: 1350–1365.

Shiner RL. A developmental perspective on personality disorders: lessons from research on normal personality development in childhood and adolescence. J Personal Disord 2005; 19: 202–210.

Skodol AE, Gunderson JG, Shea MT, McGlashan TH, Morey LC, Sanislow CA, Bender DS, Grilo CM, Zanarini MC, Yen S, Pagano ME, Stout RL. The Collaborative Longitudinal Personality Disorders Study (CLPS): overview and implications. J Personal Disord 2005; 19: 487–504.

Tackett J, Krueger RF. Interpreting personality as a vulnerability for psychopathology: a developmental approach to the personality-psychopathology relationship. In Hankin BL, Abela JRZ (eds) Development of Psychopathology: A Vulnerability-Stress Perspective. Thousand Oaks, CA: Sage, 2005, pp. 199–242.

Tyrer P. Borderline personality disorder: a motley diagnosis in need of reform. Lancet 1999; 354: 2095–2096.

Verheul R, Widiger TA. A meta-analysis of the prevalence and usage of the personality disorder not otherwise specified (PDNOS) diagnosis. J Personal Disord 2004; 18: 309–319.

Wakefield JC. The concept of mental disorder: on the boundary between biological facts and social values. Am Psychol 1992; 47: 373–388.

Westen D, Arkowitz-Westen L. Limitations of axis II in diagnosing personality pathology in clinical practice. Am J Psychiatry 1998; 155: 1767–1771.

Westen D, Gabbard GO, Blagov P. Back to the future: personality structure as a context for psychopathology. In Krueger RF, Tackett JL (eds) Personality and Psychopathology. New York: Guilford, 2006a, pp. 335–372.

Westen D, Shedler J, Bradley R. A prototype approach to personality disorder diagnosis. Am J Psychiatry 2006b; 163: 846–856.

Widiger TA, Simonsen E. Alternative dimensional models of personality disorder: finding a common ground. J Personal Disord 2005; 19: 110–130.

Widiger TA, Costa PT Jr, McCrae RR. A proposal for Axis II: diagnosing personality disorders using the five-factor model. In Costa PT Jr, Widiger TA (eds) Personality Disorders and the Five-Factor Model of Personality. Washington, DC: American Psychological Association, 2002, pp. 431–456.

Widiger TA, Simonsen E, Krueger R, Livesley JW, Verheul R. Personality disorder research agenda for the DSM-V. J Personal Disord 2005; 19: 315–338.

Widiger TA, Costa PT Jr, Samuel DB. Assessment of maladaptive personality traits. In Strack S (ed) Differentiating Normal and Abnormal Personality. New York: Springer, 2006, pp. 311–333.

# 8

# A DIMENSIONAL APPROACH TO DEVELOPMENTAL PSYCHOPATHOLOGY

James J. Hudziak, M.D.
Thomas M. Achenbach, Ph.D.
Robert R. Althoff, M.D.
Daniel S. Pine, M.D.

Multiple sources of variance affect the expression of psychopathology. In this chapter, we discuss how these sources of variance complicate both research and clinical management. We argue that these sources of variance must be considered in order to make valid, sensitive, and specific diagnoses appropriate for persons of all ages and both genders. We further argue that a quantitative axis in future DSMs will allow for adding dimensional features to DSM that can help clinicians and scientists alike evaluate not only the presence or absence of pathology but also the degree to which disorders are manifested. Equally important, dimensionalization can facilitate estimation of effect sizes in evidence-based practice and research. We point out that child psychiatrists and developmental psychologists have long used a wide variety of standardized dimensional measures in both research and clinical settings and that a significant amount of research has already been carried out re-

Reprinted with permission from Hudziak JJ, Achenbach TM, Althoff RR, Pine DS. "A Dimensional Approach to Developmental Psychopathology." *International Journal of Methods in Psychiatric Research* 2007; 16(S1): S16–S23.

lating these measures to DSM diagnoses. This work provides a foundation for dimensionalizing some aspects of DSM.

## DSM as a Categorical Taxonomy

Particularly since the major changes introduced by *Diagnostic and Statistical Manual of Mental Disorders,* Third Edition (DSM-III; American Psychiatric Association 1980), DSM has been a categorical taxonomy that has worked reasonably well for adult psychopathology. Its utility for adults may result from the fact that most research on psychopathology prior to DSM-III was done on adults. In fact, the Feighner criteria (Feighner et al. 1972), often cited as a key source of the radical changes embodied in DSM-III, essentially listed 14 categories for adult disorders. These disorders were selected because they had been sufficiently researched to engender the Robins and Guze (1970) criteria for valid psychiatric diagnosis, including clinical description, laboratory studies, delimitation from other disorders, follow-up studies, and family studies. The 14 Feighner diagnoses did not include a single child disorder. Since the publication of DSM-III, research on child psychopathology has accelerated dramatically, which has highlighted strengths and weaknesses of DSM for the developmental study of psychopathology.

Child psychopathology differs from adult psychopathology in many ways. One particularly salient difference is that the expression of psychopathology in children often changes in both magnitude and character as development progresses. Moreover, the developmental study of psychopathology must take account of age-related changes in what is considered normal and adaptive, such that behaviors considered pathological at one age may be considered normal at another age, and vice versa. Another salient difference is that assessment of psychopathology in children and adolescents requires multiple sources of information, such as parents, teachers, and children themselves. The modest agreement typically found among sources makes it hard to categorize children as sick versus well. Questions arise, for example, as to whether decisions should be based on averages across reports by multiple informants or on the most severe problems reported by any informant.

Because of these multiple sources of variance in childhood diagnosis, quantitative differences may be more crucial for child than adult diagnoses. DSM's categorical approach has proven difficult to apply to children because it fails to identify these crucial differences. To take account of developmental differences in the expression of psychopathology, a nosological system needs to take account of (1) variations in both typical and atypical behaviors across age; (2) gender differences in the expression of psychopathology; (3) differences among sources of information; and (4) tendencies for children to manifest multiple kinds of problems. Research stimulated by DSM-III, DSM-III-R (American Psychiatric Association 1987), and DSM-IV (American Psychiatric Association 1994) has contributed to developmental understanding of psychopathology and to its dimensional assessment in recent decades. It is thus a propitious time to consider adding dimensional features to DSM.

# Why Add Dimensional Features to DSM?

We propose adding dimensional features to complement the categorical aspects of DSM. The dimensional and categorical approaches each have advantages and disadvantages. The advantages of the categorical approach are detailed elsewhere in this book (see Chapter 2 by Kraemer). Disadvantages of a dimensional-only approach have also been described. These include its inconsistency with the prevailing diagnostic approach that is used by clinicians to make yes-or-no decisions about treatment. However, cut points can certainly be applied to dimensional measures as a basis for yes-or-no decisions. It has also been argued that collecting dimensional information might be more expensive than categorical information, although this is not necessarily so, because many dimensional measures can be self-administered by informants. We argue that a purely categorical approach fails to account for important sources of variance. For example, neural systems that underlie behavior differ by gender and age. Consequently, a diagnostic system must take account of gender and age variance as well as informant variance.

# Using Dimensional Approaches to Account for Multiple Sources of Variance

Over the past three decades, thousands of studies of child and adolescent psychopathology have used dimensional approaches in epidemiologic and clinical samples. Some dimensional measures, such as the Child Behavior Checklist (CBCL; Achenbach and Rescorla 2001), comprise descriptions of children's problems that were not based directly on DSM criteria, although they have been found to agree well with some DSM diagnostic categories. Other measures, such as the Conners' Rating Scales (CRS; Conners 2001) and the Behavior Assessment System for Children (Reynolds and Kamphaus 1998), include paraphrases of DSM criteria. In addition to instruments for broad clinical and epidemiologic applications, other instruments focus on narrower ranges of psychopathology, such as the Strengths and Weaknesses of ADHD-Symptoms and Normal-Behavior scale (Hay et al. 2007), the Autism Diagnostic Interview (Lord et al. 1994), the Social Responsiveness Scale (Constantino et al. 2000), the Yale-Brown Obsessive Compulsive Scale (Goodman et al. 1989), and the Young Mania Rating Scale (Young et al. 1978). These instruments (some interviews, some questionnaires) quantify the degree to which individuals manifest particular kinds of problems.

Dimensional measures of child psychopathology have become so common that teachers, pediatricians, and other non-psychiatric personnel are quite accustomed to using them. These instruments address weaknesses inherent in a one-size-fits-all system such as DSM. They provide quantitative indices of variance in symptoms and normative behavior by age and gender. Although it is beyond the scope of this chapter to compare each of the dimensional measures, suffice it to say that each has strengths and weaknesses and proponents and critics. Despite their widespread use, dimensional measures are currently orphaned from the DSM nosology. We argue that they should be more central to the assessment and care of children in order to advance evidence-based psychiatry.

# Neuroscientific and Genomic Explanations of Psychopathology May Require Quantification

In this era of neuroscience and genomics, taxonomic approaches are needed that can encompass diverse neural circuits and genes relevant to psychopathology. Developmental neurobiology research shows that the connections, anatomy, and physiology of the human brain change dramatically across development (Thompson et al. 2000), with important variations by gender (Castellanos et al. 2002) and by genetic makeup (Meyer-Lindenberg et al. 2006). Applying the current categorical taxonomy, in the absence of other approaches, has weaknesses. For example, if genetic or neural aspects of psychopathology show continuous associations with psychopathologic behaviors, the categorical approach will have less statistical power than the current taxonomic approach (Bobb et al. 2005). Moreover, genetic findings and brain imaging document overlaps among DSM categories, whereby some genes and neural factors may confer susceptibility to disorders that belong to different DSM categories, such as anxiety and depression, as opposed to narrow DSM-defined conditions. For example, in the case of neural development, a great deal is known about the amygdala's size and function, both of which vary with the age, gender, and genetic makeup of individuals (Durston et al. 2001; Walhovd et al. 2005). Consequently, disorders that may be related to the amygdala, such as conduct disorder (CD), major depressive disorder (MDD), and anxiety disorders (Sterzer et al. 2005), need to be understood in relation to age, gender, and genetic differences. A taxonomy that employs the same diagnostic rules and cut points for a 17-year-old male and a 5-year-old female may not be sensitive to underlying neural correlates of psychopathology. Brain regions such as the prefrontal cortex, implicated in developmental psychopathology, exhibit robust age-related changes in structure, function, and in the nature of associations with measures of information processing, specifically the measures of information processing that exhibit parallel changes with age. This raises questions about the degree to which changes in prefrontal cortical structure and function relate to changes in psychiatric symptoms over similar time periods. Symptom scales sensitive to developmental changes in behavior might be more sensitive to changes in the relationship between neural processes and symptoms. These considerations apply to adult and geriatric age groups as well. Our diagnostic system must allow for neural and genetic variations in order to benefit from neuroscientific and genomic advances. It must therefore be sensitive to variance related to age, gender, genes, and comorbidity.

# Sources of Variance Not Considered or Controlled for in DSM

We consider here several sources of variance that are largely ignored by the current edition of DSM but could be incorporated into future editions by dimensionalizing at least some aspects of diagnostic criteria.

## GENDER

It has long been known that three to seven times more boys than girls meet DSM diagnostic criteria for ADHD. However, in adulthood, nearly as many women as men meet DSM criteria for ADHD (3.2% versus 5.4%; Kessler et al. 2006). The reasons for the gender disparity in childhood and its disappearance in adulthood are unknown. However, a categorical approach that fails to specify gender may impede understanding of these differences. The CRS employ DSM ADHD items coupled with quantitative norms by gender, age, and informant. The CRS identify just as many girls as boys as meeting criteria for ADHD in early childhood, at least in part because gender-specific norms are used to determine which children are statistically deviant on ADHD scales (Hudziak et al. 2005b). Using DSM criteria, by contrast, girls who are significantly impaired often fail to meet the diagnostic threshold, which is the same for both genders at all ages. By slightly decreasing the number of criteria needed to meet diagnostic thresholds for girls, one would find nearly equal percentages of boys and girls with impairment in the attentional domains. Dimensional approaches provide systematic methods for selecting gender-sensitive cutoffs.

## AGE

Age is another source of variance that DSM criteria do not take into account. Those of us who treat ADHD are often reminded of the weakness of the categorical approach when we are asked to evaluate 2-, 12-, 22-, 32-, 42-, 52-, and even 62-year-old patients according to the same criteria for all ages. The neurodevelopmental level of many 2-year-olds renders them more inattentive, hyperactive, and impulsive than older children. Just 3 years later, the same children are usually more attentive, less active, and less impulsive. Some argue that developmental considerations make the DSM ADHD criteria inappropriate for preschoolers. However, the same can be said about applying the ADHD criteria to 62-year-olds. Many of us have been consulted by seniors who worry that they may have new-onset ADHD because they meet many of the DSM criteria. Although it may be possible for new ADHD symptoms to occur in older people, these people often are experiencing normative cognitive decline. When relying only on categorical approaches to taxonomy, it is difficult to incorporate multiple aspects of development into the diagnostic process. The categorical approach renders diagnoses suspect by failing to consider the remarkable changes the human brain undergoes over the course of development.

Dimensional criteria reduce the need for arbitrary decisions about transitions from one developmental period to another. Dimensional criteria also enable us to track psychopathology from childhood into adolescence and adulthood. For example, voluminous research supports a distinction between two dimensions of conduct problems in both children and adults, i.e., overt (or aggressive) versus covert (or rule-breaking) dimensions. CD symptom criteria can be easily quantified by computing symptom scores. However, these scores should be separated into at least the aggressive versus rule-breaking dimensions. Research in several countries indicates that individuals' rankings on the aggressive dimension are more stable across developmental periods and are influenced more by genetic factors than are their rankings on the rule-breaking dimension (Eley et al. 1999; Stanger et al. 1997). Child/adolescent scores for the aggressive and rule-breaking dimensions foretell differences in adult outcomes. Moreover, dividing CD symptoms into aggressive and rule-breaking dimensions avoids the arbitrary cut point of age 18 for moving from CD to antisocial personality disorder, for which 40%–50% of adolescents with CD eventually meet criteria (Steiner and Dunne 1997). A dimensional approach clearly reveals developmental continuities in aggressive and rule-breaking dimensions into adulthood rather than implying that adolescents suddenly acquire an adult disorder on their 18th birthday.

## INFORMANTS

In addition to differences by age and gender, informants are also sources of variance in diagnostic data. Although diagnostic data in child psychiatric clinics come primarily from mothers, mothers are only one of several relevant sources of data. Child psychiatrists and psychologists typically collect data from multiple informants to get more complete pictures of children. The current DSM does not provide standardized methods for incorporating data from multiple informants, despite practice parameter recommendations that data from multiple informants be routinely obtained (American Academy of Child and Adolescent Psychiatry 2007; Dulcan 1997). We know that mothers and fathers often fail to agree, that parents and teachers rarely agree, and that parent and teacher reports almost never agree with child reports (Verhulst and van der Ende 1992).

Categorical criteria greatly complicate incorporation of disparate data into the diagnostic process. For example, when a mother reports six criterial symptoms of ADHD, inattentive type with impairment, but the teacher reports only five, it is hard for the conscientious clinician to determine whether the child should be diagnosed as having ADHD. The six-symptom threshold required for a diagnosis of ADHD means that the child has the disorder according to the mother's report but not according to the teacher's report.

A dimensional approach, by contrast, would indicate 83% agreement between the mother's and teacher's reports, while also retaining the context-specific descriptors of the child. From a neuroscience and genetic research perspective, the availability of data from multiple informants enables clinicians and researchers to quantify similarities and differences in the neural and genetic correlates of behaviors recognized by parents, teachers, children, and any other informants. This raises the following question: How can we reconcile the 83% agreement between the mother and teacher in symptoms with the 0% agreement in the DSM diagnosis?

An example of a dimensional answer to this question is provided by the CBCL family of instruments. Data obtained from mothers and fathers using the CBCL, from teachers using the Teacher's Report Form, and from children using the Youth Self-Report are scored using separate norms based on national samples of each type of informant. Each informant is viewed as providing potentially valuable information about the child, as reported by that informant. Correlations between the informants' reports are displayed and are designated as above average, average, or below average on the basis of comparisons with correlations found for large reference samples of similar informants. In this way, evidence can be presented regarding the child's emotional and behavioral strengths and weaknesses in a variety of settings and from a variety of perspectives. It is not uncommon to find that mothers, fathers, teachers, and children report different problems. The clinician and researcher alike can use these data to consider variations in children's functioning and to design interventions accordingly. Additional data from repeated assessments provide evidence-based frameworks for evaluating the progress and outcomes of treatment. DSM's categorical structure and lack of normative data make it hard to deal with informant variance.

## COMORBIDITY

Some children who meet DSM criteria for ADHD also meet criteria for oppositional defiant disorder (ODD) and MDD. Such children are said to suffer from comorbidity, or the co-occurrence of multiple disorders. Many studies have shown that most children with ADHD also meet diagnostic criteria for other disorders (Faraone et al. 2001). Children who suffer from the constellation of ADHD, ODD, and MDD are often diagnosed as having a broad phenotype of juvenile bipolar disorder (JBD), meaning that criteria are not met for the narrow DSM-IV definition of bipolar affective disorder (Althoff et al. 2006; Faraone et al. 2005). Dimensional approaches show that these children have a condition that is genetically distinct from ADHD, ODD, or MDD. In other words, they may suffer from a single disorder (Hudziak et al. 2005a) rather than three comorbid disorders. Just what the disorder is, no one knows for sure. Leibenluft and colleagues (Brotman et al. 2006) have suggested that the condition be called severe mood dysregulation. There is no clear agreement on how best to characterize these children in terms of DSM categories.

Using a CBCL–JBD profile, our group has shown that children with this phenotype have some of the highest endorsement rates for suicidal behavior of any clinical group (Althoff et al. 2006). Despite the lack of agreement about how to fit these children into DSM categories, there are recommendations, at least in the United States, to treat them with therapies tested only for narrow-spectrum bipolar disorder (American Academy of Child and Adolescent Psychiatry 2007). Specifically, these children are treated with medications that have been tested only on children with narrow-spectrum bipolar disorders, if they are tested on children at all. Although it is not known what the best treatment would be, the lack of a clear phenotypic definition makes it unlikely that appropriate clinical trials of this highly morbid and potentially lethal disorder will be done soon. This is an example of how a categorical system that represents higher order patterns in terms of comorbidity among separate disorders may impede treatment decisions (American Academy of Child and Adolescent Psychiatry 2007; Kowatch et al. 2005). A dimensional approach can advance our knowledge of complex conditions by reframing comorbidity in terms of higher order patterns.

## Putting It All Together: The Example of Conduct Disorder

To summarize, we use CD to demonstrate the need for a dimensional characterization of developmental psychopathology. CD provides a classic example of differences between the current DSM approach and dimensional approaches. As shown in Table 8–1, DSM-IV specifies 15 symptoms for CD. The diagnostic rules state that children who have at least three CD symptoms, plus impairment, meet criteria for CD. An 11-year-old girl who skips school, stays out after curfew, and has shoplifted thus has CD. So does a 17-year-old boy who has all 15 symptoms, including using a weapon, cruelty to animals and people, stealing while confronting a victim, and forced sex. An 11-year-old girl who has only skipped school and shoplifted would not meet criteria for CD. Thus, the two 11-year-old girls are categorically different from each other, but one is categorically like the 17-year-old

---

**TABLE 8–1.** DSM-IV diagnostic criteria for conduct disorder

---

A. A repetitive and persistent pattern of behavior in which the basic rights of others or major age-appropriate societal norms or rules are violated, as manifested by the presence of three (or more) of the following criteria in the past 12 months, with at least one criterion present in the past 6 months:

Aggression to people and animals

1. Often bullies, threatens, or intimidates others.

2. Often initiates physical fights.

3. Has used a weapon that can cause serious physical harm to others (e.g., a bat, brick, broken bottle, knife, gun).

4. Has been physically cruel to people.

5. Has been physically cruel to animals.

6. Has stolen while confronting a victim (e.g., mugging, purse snatching, extortion, armed robbery).

7. Has forced someone into sexual activity.

**Destruction of property**

8. Has deliberately engaged in fire setting with the intention of causing serious damage.

9. Has deliberately destroyed others' property (other than by fire setting).

**Deceitfulness or theft**

10. Has broken into someone else's house, building, or car.

11. Often lies to obtain goods or favors or to avoid obligations (i.e., "cons" others).

12. Has stolen items of nontrivial value without confronting a victim (e.g., shoplifting, but without breaking and entering; forgery).

**Serious violations of rules**

13. Often stays out at night despite parental prohibitions, beginning before age 13 years.

14. Has run away from home overnight at least twice while living in a parental or parental surrogate home (or once without returning for a lengthy period).

15. Is often truant from school, beginning before age 13 years.

B. The disturbance in behavior causes clinically significant impairment in social, academic, or occupational functioning.

C. If the individual is 18 years or older, criteria are not met for antisocial personality disorder.

---

*Source.* Reprinted from American Psychiatric Association 1994. Used with permission.

boy. This categorical confound illustrates the difficulties in applying DSM criteria to children and adolescents.

The categorical criteria do not take account of differences in the degrees to which children and adolescents manifest criterial symptoms (e.g., 2/15 symptoms versus 3/15 symptoms versus 15/15 symptoms). They also fail to reflect developmental differences (in this case age 11 versus 17) as well as gender differences. Lastly, they do not take account of informant differences in reports for each child and also in the differential relevance of different informants' reports for particular kinds of problems, boys versus girls, and different ages. For all these reasons, it is difficult to conceptualize data on CD using the DSM approach in relation to age, gender, informant, and quantitative differences.

When using a dimensional approach to conduct problems, we find that children with ODD or CD can be described in terms of dimensions such as those embodied in the aggressive behavior and rule-breaking behavior syndromes identified and assessed by the CBCL family of instruments. Using this approach, we can evaluate children on dimensions in relation to national norms that include informant, age, and gender variance. The dimensions and norms extend into adulthood, providing continuity in the evaluation of the 17-year-old boy when he reaches age 18, without necessitating a new diagnosis that implies a change of psychopathology on his 18th birthday.

# A Proposal for How Categorical and Dimensional Approaches Can Be Further Developed Together

In child and adolescent psychiatry and psychology, there is at least as much research on dimensional approaches as on categorical approaches. Given the abundance of dimensional data, it seems feasible to incorporate provisions for variance related to age, gender, and informant into diagnostic criteria. Clearly, clinicians and researchers need cut points in order to make decisions about treatment and about inclusion in clinical trials. In a dimensional system, such cut points can be adjusted according to the different sources of variance. Dimensional data can then provide age-, gender-, and informant-specific starting points for treatment studies, longitudinal studies, and outcome studies. The addition of dimensional data could then lead to iterative improvement in categorical rules for treatment decisions.

It has long been held that dimensional approaches are less useful clinically. We envision a synergistic system that allows a categorical descriptor, e.g., ADHD, and a dimensional profile, e.g., the degree to which a child suffers from deviance in attention problems, aggressive behavior, and anxious/depressed problems. This dimensional profile can then be used in evidence-based approaches to determine not only whether the child's categorical state changes (e.g., the child no longer has

ADHD) but also to what degree the core symptoms (attention problems) and associated symptoms (aggression and anxious depression) change (either diminish or, as we have seen in many cases, increase in intensity). Because this "clinical application" of a combined approach provides gender, developmental, and informant sensitivity, we can determine whether the child's improvement or worsening varies by setting. By combining categorical and quantitative approaches, we can more fully utilize evidence-based approaches in child psychiatry.

## Conclusions

Dimensional approaches are already commonly used in child psychiatry and psychology. We presented examples of ADHD and CD where there is clear support for a dimensional approach. Similar support exists for dimensional approaches to childhood anxiety, depression, and autistic spectrum disorders. The advantages of dimensional approaches include the ability to generate quantitative profiles that cut across common psychopathologies. These profiles present psychopathology in terms that are both sensitive and specific in relation to gender and age variance. Dimensional approaches offer many advantages for neuroscience and genomics. It has been argued that we may identify continua for some kinds of psychopathology and categories for other kinds. For these reasons, we have argued for a complementary system that includes both approaches. We note that dimensional approaches are needed in order to inculcate potentially useful endophenotypic and genetic discoveries into our assessment procedures and that our taxonomy should facilitate rather than impede the advance of knowledge. Dimensional approaches are thus needed to characterize psychopathologies, to search for their underlying genetic and neural mechanisms, and to discover treatments and cures.

## References

Achenbach T, Rescorla L. Manual for the ASEBA School-Age Forms & Profiles. Burlington, VT: University of Vermont Research Center for Children, Youth, and Families, 2001.

Althoff RR, Rettew DC, Faraone SV, Boomsma DI, Hudziak JJ. Latent class analysis shows strong heritability of the Child Behavior Checklist-juvenile bipolar phenotype. Biol Psychiatry 2006; 60(9): 903–911.

American Academy of Child and Adolescent Psychiatry. Practice parameter for the assessment and treatment of children and adolescents with bipolar disorder. J Am Acad Child Adolesc Psychiatry 2007; 46(1): 107–125.

American Psychiatric Association. Diagnostic and Statistical Manual of Mental Disorders, 3rd Edition. Washington, DC: American Psychiatric Association, 1980.

American Psychiatric Association. Diagnostic and Statistical Manual of Mental Disorders, 3rd Edition, Revised. Washington, DC: American Psychiatric Association, 1987.

American Psychiatric Association. Diagnostic and Statistical Manual of Mental Disorders, 4th Edition. Washington, DC: American Psychiatric Association, 1994.

Bobb AJ, Castellanos FX, Addington AM, Rapoport JL. Molecular genetic studies of ADHD: 1991 to 2004. Am J Med Genet B Neuropsychiatr Genet 2005; 132(1): 109–125.

Brotman MA, Schmajuk M, Rich BA, et al. Prevalence, clinical correlates, and longitudinal course of severe mood dysregulation in children. Biol Psychiatry 2006; 60(9): 991–997.

Castellanos FX, Lee PP, Sharp W, et al. Developmental trajectories of brain volume abnormalities in children and adolescents with attention-deficit/hyperactivity disorder. JAMA 2002; 288(14): 1740–1748.

Conners C. Conners' Rating Scales—Revised. New York: Multi-Health Systems, 2001.

Constantino JN, Przybeck T, Friesen D, Todd RD. Reciprocal social behavior in children with and without pervasive developmental disorders. J Dev Behav Pediatr 2000; 21(1): 2–11.

Dulcan M. Practice parameters for the assessment and treatment of children, adolescents, and adults with attention-deficit/hyperactivity disorder. American Academy of Child and Adolescent Psychiatry. J Am Acad Child Adolesc Psychiatry 1997; 36(10 Suppl): 85S–121S.

Durston S, Hulshoff Pol HE, Casey BJ, Giedd JN, Buitelaar JK, van Engeland H. Anatomical MRI of the developing human brain: what have we learned? J Am Acad Child Adolesc Psychiatry 2001; 40(9): 1012–1020.

Eley TC, Lichtenstein P, Stevenson J. Sex differences in the etiology of aggressive and nonaggressive antisocial behavior: results from two twin studies. Child Dev 1999; 70(1): 155–168.

Faraone SV, Biederman J, Mick E, et al. A family study of psychiatric comorbidity in girls and boys with attention-deficit/hyperactivity disorder. Biol Psychiatry 2001; 50(8): 586–592.

Faraone SV, Althoff RR, Hudziak JJ, Monuteaux M, Biederman J. The CBCL predicts DSM bipolar disorder in children: a receiver operating characteristic curve analysis. Bipolar Disord 2005; 7(6): 518–524.

Feighner JP, Robins E, Guze SB, Woodruff RA Jr, Winokur G, Munoz R. Diagnostic criteria for use in psychiatric research. Arch Gen Psychiatry 1972; 26(1): 57–63.

Goodman WK, Price LH, Rasmussen SA, et al. The Yale–Brown Obsessive Compulsive Scale. I. Development, use, and reliability. Arch Gen Psychiatry 1989; 46(11): 1006–1011.

Hay DA, Bennett KS, Levy F, Sergeant J, Swanson J. A twin study of attention-deficit/hyperactivity disorder dimensions rated by the Strengths and Weaknesses of ADHD-Symptoms and Normal-Behavior (SWAN) scale. Biol Psychiatry 2007; 61(5): 700–705.

Hudziak JJ, Althoff RR, Derks EM, Faraone SV, Boomsma DI. Prevalence and genetic architecture of Child Behavior Checklist-juvenile bipolar disorder. Biol Psychiatry 2005a; 58(7): 562–568.

Hudziak JJ, Derks EM, Althoff RR, Rettew DC, Boomsma DI. The genetic and environmental contributions to attention deficit hyperactivity disorder as measured by the Conners' Rating Scales—Revised. Am J Psychiatry 2005b; 162(9): 1614–1620.

Kessler RC, Adler L, Barkley R, et al. The prevalence and correlates of adult ADHD in the United States: results from the National Comorbidity Survey Replication. Am J Psychiatry 2006; 163(4): 716–723.

Kowatch RA, Fristad M, Birmaher B, Wagner KD, Findling RL, Hellander M. Treatment guidelines for children and adolescents with bipolar disorder. J Am Acad Child Adolesc Psychiatry 2005; 44(3): 213–235.

Lord C, Rutter M, Le Couteur A. Autism Diagnostic Interview—Revised: a revised version of a diagnostic interview for caregivers of individuals with possible pervasive developmental disorders. J Autism Dev Disord 1994; 24(5): 659–685.

Meyer-Lindenberg A, Nichols T, Callicott JH, et al. Impact of complex genetic variation in COMT on human brain function. Mol Psychiatry 2006; 11(9): 867–877, 797.

Reynolds C, Kamphaus R. Behavior Assessment System for Children Manual, 2nd Edition. Circle Pines, MN: American Guidance Service, 1998.

Robins E, Guze SB. Establishment of diagnostic validity in psychiatric illness: its application to schizophrenia. Am J Psychiatry 1970; 126(7): 983–987.

Stanger C, Achenbach T, Verhulst F. Accelerated longitudinal comparisons of aggressive versus delinquent syndromes. Dev Psychopathol 1997; 9(1): 43–58.

Steiner H, Dunne J. Summary of the practice parameters for the assessment and treatment of children and adolescents with conduct disorder. J Am Acad Child Adolesc Psychiatry 1997; 36(10): 1482–1485.

Sterzer P, Stadler C, Krebs A, Kleinschmidt A, Poustka F. Abnormal neural responses to emotional visual stimuli in adolescents with conduct disorder. Biol Psychiatry 2005; 57(1): 7–15.

Thompson PM, Giedd JN, Woods RP, MacDonald D, Evans AC, Toga AW. Growth patterns in the developing brain detected by using continuum mechanical tensor maps. Nature 2000; 404(6774): 190–193.

Verhulst FC, van der Ende J. Agreement between parents' reports and adolescents' self-reports of problem behavior. J Child Psychol Psychiatry 1992; 33(6): 1011–1023.

Walhovd KB, Fjell AM, Reinvang I, et al. Effects of age on volumes of cortex, white matter and subcortical structures. Neurobiol Aging 2005; 26(9): 1261–1270, discussion 1275–1278.

Young RC, Biggs JT, Ziegler VE, Meyer DA. A rating scale for mania: reliability, validity and sensitivity. Br J Psychiatry 1978; 133: 429–435.

# 9

# DIMENSIONAL OPTIONS FOR DSM-V: THE WAY FORWARD

John E. Helzer, M.D.
Hans-Ulrich Wittchen, Ph.D.
Robert F. Krueger, Ph.D.
Helena Chmura Kraemer, Ph.D.

The creation of explicit categorical definitions for the diagnosis of mental disorders in DSM-III, published by the American Psychiatric Association (APA) in 1980, represented a major shift in the classification of mental illness. The positive consequences of this achievement for both the clinical practice and the science of mental disorders have been vast. But scientific progress, fostered in part by DSM over the past quarter century, has significantly increased awareness of the limitations of categorical definitions of mental illnesses. Taxonomic experts, including many of those on the DSM Task Forces, have been well aware of the limitations of exclusively categorical diagnostic criteria. A fundamental taxonomic quandary, as highlighted by Darrel Regier in his foreword to this volume, is how to define categorical entities given the possibility that "disorders might merge into one another with no natural boundary in between" (Kendell and Jablensky 2003). A related issue is the need to reconcile the clinical use of diagnostic cut-points that also identify individuals in the general population who are sufficiently impaired to require treatment. These problems have not been addressed on the basis of careful scientific exploration, and they now complicate the work of the newly appointed DSM-V Task Force. Other fundamental issues facing the Task Force and the

DSM-V diagnostic workgroups include the high level of comorbidity across the illness entities defined by DSM, and the need to create a taxonomy that is developmentally, culturally, and gender sensitive. As will be summarized in this chapter, these issues and others are taken up by one or more of the authors in this volume. As these chapters demonstrate, a supplementary dimensional approach to diagnosis could shed new light on all of the above taxonomic issues.

This book is essentially the proceedings from the conference "Dimensional Approaches to Diagnostic Classification: A Critical Appraisal," held in July 2006. This effort was one in a series of international conferences titled "Refining the Research Agenda for DSM-V" that is described in the Foreword. The previous chapters of this volume reflect the discussions and recommendations regarding the use of dimensional approaches for selected diagnoses. This chapter, written by the conference co-chairs, summarizes those presentations and organizes them into a set of suggestions for developing dimensional alternatives for DSM-V categorical diagnoses.

## Considerations for Dimensional Assessment

The agenda of this conference was not to replace categorical diagnoses in DSM-V, but rather to consider ways by which the addition of continuous, "dimensional" measures into the various diagnostic domains might help resolve some of the critical taxonomic issues currently facing the field of mental health. The intention was to consider supplementary dimensional approaches to the categorical definitions that would also relate back to the categorical definitions in an unambiguous way. It was overtly recognized that both categorical and dimensional approaches to diagnosis are important both for clinical work and for research, and that the ideal taxonomy would offer both. However, it was also recognized that in order to avoid diagnostic chaos, the dimensional scale must reflect the categorical definition and that the two must have a clear and obvious relationship to one another.

In Chapter 2, Helena Chmura Kraemer lays out the rationale and multiple advantages of having both categorical and dimensional diagnostic options in DSM-V. Apropos of a dimensional approach, Kraemer notes that within each diagnostic entity there are multiple options for creating a continuous measure (a dimensional scale) based on a categorical definition. These options include the number of symptoms, severity or duration of symptoms, level of illness impairment, and others. Basing a dimension on those variables representing the most clinically important sources of heterogeneity for each diagnosis would optimize dimensional utility in a way that is diagnosis-specific. However, a drawback of an approach that is unique to each diagnosis is the likelihood of considerable variation across diagnoses in how the dimensions are constructed, potentially even within the same group of diagnoses. Thus, if dimensional options for the categorical diagnoses are adopted, a major question for the DSM-V Task Force is whether to 1) encourage each workgroup to create dimensional approaches that are most appropriate to the diagnoses they are defining; or 2) opt for a dimensional framework that is more consistent across diagnoses.

## Some Options for Dimensional Equivalents

In Chapter 3, Helzer and colleagues offer an option for a dimensional equivalent for the diagnosis of substance dependence that provides a degree of interdiagnostic flexibility but also cross-diagnostic consistency, and in a way that would minimally impact response burden. In this proposal, the diagnostic workgroup first creates the categorical definition and sets the diagnostic threshold, just as in previous versions of DSM. It is then suggested that dimensionality begin at the symptom level, with each symptom being scored on a 3-point scale, rather than dichotomously as in the past. Anchors for the 3-point scale could vary depending on the specific symptom. Using DSM-IV symptoms as examples, Helzer et al. note that substance withdrawal might logically be scored in terms of severity: none (never occurred), mild (has occurred but never severe), or severe. A symptom such as "sacrificing other activities in order to use a substance" might be more logically scored in terms of its frequency: never, sometimes, frequent. Both correspond to a simple numerical scale of 0, 1, or 2. The authors then propose the selection of an appropriate statistical methodology to create the dimensional scale based on scored symptoms—for example, using multiple logistic regression with the categorical diagnosis as the dependent variable to identify the dimensional score that most closely corresponds to the categorical threshold as originally set by the workgroup. Since it begins with the defined DSM-V criteria, this method for creating dimensional equivalents could be used for all DSM-V definitions. The principal advantage of this proposal is the consistent and obvious relationship between the categorical and dimensional definitions. Another advantage is that the same clinical information is used for both the categorical and the dimensional diagnosis. This approach optimizes efficiency of data collection for both clinicians and investigators. It also optimizes efficiency for the patients since it permits both categorical and dimensional assesssment with virtually no increase in response burden. If we assume the diagnostic criteria reflect the workgroup's best judgment about the variables most clinically relevant to that diagnosis, this also meets Kraemer's recommendation that the dimensional scale be based on "those variables representing the most clinically important sources of heterogeneity." However, this proposal does not allow for the inclusion of nondiagnostic variables, such as biological tests, in the dimensional scale unless they are a part of the diagnostic criteria.

Acknowledging the dimensional nature of depressive disorders, Andrews and colleagues offer another interesting option to utilize scales that are already in existence for quantifying categorical diagnoses (see Chapter 4). The particular example they give is the Patient Health Questionnaire (PHQ-9; Spitzer et al. 2000) for quantifying current (past 2 weeks) major depression. This approach would benefit from any existing studies of reliability and validity of the chosen scale. In addition, many such scales have been designed to be self-administered, and questionionable wording has been refined to ensure the items are comprehendible. There are also disadvantages. One, noted by Andrews et al., is that any single existing scale may not be sufficiently comprehensive to cover all the diagnoses within a diagnostic group (e.g., all the affective disorders), particularly since the process of creating DSM-V will presumably result in new illness definitions such that any existing scale would have to be re-designed and re-tested. Shear et al. note in Chapter 6 that another problem is the multiple candidate scales that exist for any set of diagnoses. They estimate that hundreds of psychometric scales have been developed to measure the many domains of relevance in the anxiety disorders, including anxiety reaction, avoidance, anticipatory anxiety, worrying, and others. If existing scales were to be used, choices would have to be made among this multitude of options.

One consideration might be to develop diagnostic interviews corresponding to the new illness definitions as part of the DSM-V process. Despite the use of explicit criteria, it is often difficult to compare diagnostic results across studies because of differences in the assessment tools used to evaluate those criteria. If the DSM-V process were to result not only in new illness definitions but also the assessment instrument(s) appropriate to those definitions, cross-study consistency could be greatly improved. The DSM imprimatur on a specific diagnostic interview might enable it to become the standard for the field, just as the DSM-III diagnostic criteria have been since 1980. Comparability of results would likely serve as a strong motive for use. As Allardyce et al. note in this volume (see Chapter 5), "Symptom rating scales are now used routinely in clinical settings to monitor treatment response and relapse and to assess remission. The introduction of a formal dimensional measure in the (DSM-V) classification system would, hopefully, coordinate and optimize this use."

## Cross-Cutting Dimensions

So far, this summary has focused on measurement of specific diagnostic entities. Another topic discussed extensively at the conference was of higher order dimensions that cut across diagnoses. Shear et al. (see Chapter 6) note that the definition of panic attack, independent of any specific disorder in DSM-IV, offers a useful example of a cross-cutting concept. Its importance is confirmed by the fact that panic has now been shown to be a reliable marker of greater severity and reduced treatment responsiveness across other disorders (Bittner et al. 2004).

Both Shear et al., in the anxiety disorders (Chapter 6), and Allardyce et al., for the psychoses (Chapter 5), emphasize the importance of considering a cross-cutting taxonomic organization in DSM-V. Allardyce et al. note the coexistence of positive, negative, and disorganized factors in psychosis. Factor analytic solutions for the classification of the psychoses are more robust if they also include manic and depressive symptoms (van Os et al. 1996). There is also considerable evidence of an etio-pathological continuum across schizophrenia, schizoaffective disorder, and affective illness dating back at least a century, illustrating the prognostic significance of prominent affective symptoms in psychotic illness. This is reflected in more recent evidence supporting a biological continuum (Green et al. 2005). As Allardyce et al. note (see Chapter 5), "[Cross-cutting] dimensions across all psychotic and major affective disorders potentially could be more informative than a system where categorical diagnoses are kept artificially dimension-specific."

Hudziak et al. (Chapter 8) mention the example of children who have symptoms of attentiondeficit hyperactivity disorder (ADHD), oppositional defiant disorder (ODD), and manic depressive disorder (MDD). These children are often said to suffer from comorbidity of all three disorders. In fact, this broad panoply of symptoms appears to form a unique, cross-cutting profile that is identifiable with dimensional tools and highly heritable (Althoff et al. 2006). This example helps to show how a cross-cutting dimensional approach can actually simplify the clinical conceptualization of an illness state that is quite convoluted when relying strictly on categorical criteria.

## Taxonomic Consideration of Development, Gender, and Culture

Child and adolescent disorders also highlight the need for developmental and gender sensitivity in the taxonomy of mental disorders. In Chapter 8, Hudziak et al. point out that up to seven times as many boys as girls meet DSM diagnostic criteria for ADHD, but that in adulthood this ratio is closer to 1.5:1. This discrepancy may be largely a consequence of a lack of developmental sensitivity in DSM. Dimensional approaches, such as the Conners' Rating Scale (CRS; Connors 2001), do not confirm such a disparity in childhood because, according to Hudziak et al., "gender-specific norms are used to determine which children are statistically deviant on ADHD scales." Furthermore, dividing conduct disorder symptoms into separate aggressive and rule-breaking dimensions enables much stronger predictions of adult outcomes. Dimensional approaches also avoid the necessity of an abrupt change in diagnosis from conduct disorder to antisocial personality disorder at age 18, a categorical quirk that masks developmental changes that are actually continuous.

Sensitivity to individual characteristics, developmental plasticity, and potential diagnostic bias are more straightforward with a dimensional compared to a categorical approach. A categorical system defines a single threshold. But there is meaningful clinical variation both above and below that threshold, some of which is of developmental relevance. With a dimensional system, rather it being assumed, as DSM-IV now does, that all children who meet 3 of 15 CD criteria are alike in some important clinical respect (i.e., have conduct disorder), children can be evaluated on a dimensional scale that is nationally normed based on age, gender, ethnicity, and even, when appropriate, type of informant.

Sensitivity to similarities as well as differences is also important and may be relevant in comparing, for example, ethnicities across differing cultures. Categorical definitions can complicate cross-national comparisons of illness prevalence. It has been shown that in surveys of general populations, positive cases tend to concentrate at the categorical threshold (Helzer et al. 1985). Since one symptom can change diagnostic status, subtle differences in survey method, interview translation, or cultural response effects of even one or two relevant items can result in large differences in the estimated prevalences when defined categorically. Dimensional scales in which the full range of symptoms is considered for every case are much less vulnerable to differing prevalence caused by such variations. Thus dimensions increase the likelihood of recognizing continuities within and across large populations, when they exist.

Allardyce et al. (Chapter 5) note another potential difficulty with categorically based population prevalences. There is evidence of a continuous distribution of positive symptoms of psychosis in the general population. By identifying some point on that continuum as the illness threshold, a categorical definition creates a discontinuity that may not exist. Furthermore, our clinical conceptualization of psychosis, on which the categorical definition is based, may be biased since it is heavily weighted by those cases coming to medical attention.

## Relevance of Dimensions to Clinicians

It is sometimes claimed that while a dimensional approach may be important for researchers, it would be problematic for clinicians. This claim can be challenged on three grounds. The first challenge was forcefully articulated by Dr. Harold Eist, a clinician and former APA president, during a symposium on DSM-V at the 2006 APA annual meeting. Dr. Eist pointed out that he uses dimensions daily in his clinical practice: once a categorical diagnosis has been made, he and other clinicians must think dimensionally about severity of illness, how aggressively to treat, level of treatment response, and so forth. To paraphrase his comments, "it is a clinical necessity to think dimensionally, but we all do it differently because DSM has never provided us any guidelines." There is evidence that, when given the opportunity, clinicians will use an established dimensional tool in their clinical decision making and that such information often leads to adjustments or changes in therapy (see Chapter 4). Trivedi et al. (2006) call for routine clinical use of dimensional tools as a foundation for measurement-based care for mental disorders.

Illness staging based on dimensional assessment is routinely used clinically for diabetes mellitus and its vascular complications (Haffner 2006).

A second, and perhaps the most important, challenge to the claim of opposing research and clinical utility is that dimensions and categories are not necessarily mutually exclusive, but can be synergistic. The comments of Shear et al. in Chapter 6 highlight the issue nicely: "replacing categorical diagnostic criteria with dimensional assessment would not serve the field well....[DSM] supplies simple, reliable rules for categorical assignments required for clinical and research purposes [and] the link to a very large body of...empirical data." Thus the focus of this conference was not only on dimensional approaches but also on how to integrate them with categorical definitions, which remain vital to DSM. As Kraemer writes, "What is being proposed for DSM-V is not to substitute dimensional scales for categorical diagnoses, but to add a dimensional option to the usual categorical diagnoses for DSM-V" (emphasis added; see Chapter 2). But, it is crucial that the categorical and dimensional approaches correspond well and that the link be clear and understandable.

Finally, the claim of exclusive research utility of dimensions is also challenged by the recognition that research, by improving our understanding of illness processes and facilitating discovery of new treatments, is vitally important to our work as clinicians. Any revision to DSM, such as dimensional equivalents for the categorical diagnoses, that renders research efforts more effective and communication of research findings more precise benefits us all: practitioners, investigators, and our patients.

# Dimensional Options for DSM-V

While each of the chapters in this volume offers ideas about dimensional approaches, Shear et al. (Chapter 6) provide a useful conceptual summary by articulating three generic approaches: 1) continuous assessment of core diagnostic features as they will eventually be defined in the DSM-V criteria; 2) cross-cutting approaches; and 3) higher order factor analytic approaches. In an earlier section of this chapter, two specific options were suggested for the first approach: to utilize existing rating scales (see Chapter 4), and to create scales based directly on the new DSM-V criterion items (see Chapter 8). There was general agreement among the conferees that symptom severity is a logical basis for the "continuous assessment of core diagnostic features."

The second generic approach, cross-cutting dimensions, is not mutually exclusive with a continuous assessment of core diagnostic features. Cross-cutting approaches can be explored by selectively combining core features from more than one diagnosis (e.g., combinations of psychotic and affective symptoms) and testing them against traditional validators such as ability to predict outcome. Dimensional scoring of individual criteria within a diagnosis facilitates the assessment of cross-cutting features, just as it enhances assessment of the individual diagnoses. Even a simple quantitative measure of symptoms (e.g., 0, 1, 2) adds power for both efforts.

The third generic approach, higher order factor analytic scales, does represent a major change from how DSM has been constructed in the past. As discussed in the next section, a higher order factor analytic approach to diagnosis is an example of what is often called a "bottom-up" diagnostic process.

## Top-Down Versus Bottom-Up Approaches to Diagnosis

DSM has always been constructed in a "top-down" fashion. Within each diagnostic area, expert clinicians (the diagnostic workgroups) consult their own experience, the existing literature, and new data in order to define both the specific criterion items and the number and/or pattern of items required for a diagnosis. In contrast, a "bottom-up" system is driven primarily by empirical analysis: a large body of symptom data is collected from respondents in the general population, and statistical analysis is used to determine which symptoms cluster together into syndromes. In both designs, diagnoses can be defined categorically and/or scored dimensionally. The Childhood Behavioral Checklist (CBCL; Achenbach 1999), as discussed in Chapter 8, is an example of a dimensionally scored, bottom-up diagnostic system. Recent research has explored the relationship between DSM-IV diagnostic categories and comparable CBCL dimensions (Achenbach et al. 2005). The spectrum project (Cassano et al. 2004; Frank et al. 1998; Maser and Akiskal 2002) is an example of a bottom-up enhancement of DSM-IV for adult diagnoses.

The principal advantage of a top-down approach is its correspondence with clinical observation. The syndromal definitions are created by clinicians based on their clinical experience and relevant research findings, and the salience of the definitions to clinical work is immediately obvious. This facilitates clinical communication and diagnostic reliability. The potential weakness is that to the extent we impose our own preconceived ideas into the diagnostic definitions, the top-down approach ceases to be an empirical process. Judgments about what constitutes the core clinical criteria for a specific diagnosis differ, even among experts. Furthermore, as noted by Allardyce et al. in Chapter 5, our clinical experience tends to be biased, since those patients who come to our attention as clinicians are generally the more seriously ill and are not necessarily representative of the entire spectrum of a disorder. Explicit categorical definitions based on careful clinical observation tend to be reliable, but imposing our own preconceptions on nature may constrain validity.

A bottom-up approach is an empirical search for syndromes as they appear in the data. Clinical observation has always been important in taxonomic exploration, and conference attendees did not advocate abandoning the top-down approach in DSM-V. A more evolutionary option would be to structure DSM-V in a way that makes it possible to explore and compare top-down and bottom-up approaches, so that we could capitalize on both to improve diagnostic validity. A relevant example is provided by Krueger et al. in Chapter 7. They discuss the advantages of having core descriptive personality features as part of DSM-V, thereby reducing the large number of current Axis II symptoms to a more manageable set of core traits. These features could be created in an empirical, bottom-up manner and could inform the conception of personality and personality disorder in DSM-V. The dimensions conference generated some ideas for implementation of this evolutionary process, as discussed in the next section.

## A Simple Proposal for a Dimensional Option in DSM-V

This section begins with the presumption that the structure of DSM-V and its creation will be much like its predecessors, namely, diagnostic workgroups composed of experts from the field will decide which criterion items to include for each diagnosis, and will specify categorical thresholds. On the basis of that assumption, we suggest, in what follows, a method for creating dimensional equivalents that are linked to the categorical definitions in a way that is clearly understandable and does not increase response burden for either the clinician or the patient. In addition, we put forth a means for creating an expanded dataset that would permit systematic comparison of top-down and bottom-up approaches to diagnosis and could inform subsequent iterations of DSM. This design would permit exploration of all three generic approaches to diagnosis described in Chapter 6—core criteria, cross-cutting dimensions, and hybrid models—and would allow for gender, developmental, and cultural sensitivity.

In this proposal, the initial step is for the diagnostic workgroups to proceed as they always have in creating the phenomenological definitions for DSM, including the signs and symptoms to be ascertained and the number/pattern of these items necessary for the categorical diagnosis. The next step would be for the workgroups to specify a simple severity scale for each criterion item. In the past, a minimal severity threshold has often been implied or defined for specific symptoms. The difference here would be to make the threshold more explicit by scoring each symptom on a simple dimension. As an example, Helzer et al. propose a 3-point severity scale (0, 1, 2) for each of the substance use disorder criterion items, and such a straightforward scale could work for all diagnoses. It would seem advantageous for patients and clinicians alike if symptoms were scored in a consistent manner across diagnoses. But that decision would have to be made by each workgroup and/or the DSM-V Task Force.

While scoring symptom severity is not a necessary step, we consider it desirable for two reasons. First, even a simple 3-point specification of severity at the symptom level significantly enhances the power of dimensionality at the diagnostic level. Second, clinicians intuitively recognize the necessity of evaluating the severity of each symptom a patient reports during an examination. The suggestion here is to provide measurement guidelines in the interest of adding greater uniformity to this intuitive process. Future research would also benefit from recording symptom severity—for example, gene expression in behavioral disorders may occur at the symptom level (van Praag 1990).

The next step is to utilize appropriate statistical tools to define a dimensional scale for each diagnosis, based on the criterion items. Simply adding the number of criterion items a given patient endorses as positive is one method of scaling but is not advisable. Often two or more symptoms are highly intercorrelated; adding them can overemphasize the underlying construct they measure. Some symptoms may be inconsistent measures, and adding them in with equal weight would only introduce "noise."

Once the dimensional scale for the diagnosis has been created statistically, the final step would be to use another statistical tool to identify the scale score that most closely corresponds to the categorical diagnostic threshold as defined by the workgroup. As Helzer et al. note in Chapter 3, "An estimate of the score that best relates to the categorical diagnosis helps orient clinicians and investigators, and helps ensure concordance between the categorical and dimensional options." Selecting the appropriate statistical tool(s) for creating a dimensional scale and relating them back to categorical definition requires special expertise (Kiernan et al. 2001; Kraemer 1992). As part of the DSM-V process, steps are being taken to ensure that statistical consultation will be available to the diagnostic workgroups.

In summary, the proposal described above suggests a method for creating dimensional scaling for each diagnosis that is simple, preserves the traditional DSM workgroup function, does not increase the ascertainment burden for physicians or the response burden for patients, and bears a clear relationship to the categorical definition at both the criterion and the diagnostic level. As such, it would be a significant step forward, enhancing both clinical and scientific progress in psychiatry, and ensuring that DSM remains a vibrant, cutting-edge tool for the future. In the next section we offer a suggestion for structuring DSM-V so that it also anticipates possible needs for DSM-VI.

# Structuring DSM-V to Meet Diagnostic Needs in DSM-VI

The proposal put forth in the previous section envisions that DSM-V will be created in the traditional top-down manner. Opportunities for exploring bottom-up approaches to diagnosis, as described earlier can also be created. Any exploration or use of bottom-up approaches would be entirely optional, but conferees felt it is important to take steps now to make future systematic exploration possible. The principal advantage of a bottom-up definitional option is that it permits a more complete probe of the underlying "latent" structure of disorders. As noted earlier, in a top-down system we tend to impose our own clinical observations onto nature in order to create a common diagnostic vocabulary. In a bottom-up approach we use an empirical process to discern deviations from normality (i.e., putative disorder). The two approaches can then be compared to determine which one generates more valid diagnoses (Kendler 1990; Robins and Guze 1970).

Exploration of bottom-up approaches requires a more inclusive set of symptoms than those specified in the categorical criteria. However, the process of creating the categorical criteria in DSM actually involves consideration of a wide range of illness manifestations. Each diagnostic workgroup goes through an intellectual process of consulting the empirical data and their own clinical experience to decide which of many possible symptoms to include in the categorical criteria. In a bottom-up procedure, the selection of symptoms is done statistically. Therefore, the only step requried for a more systematic exploration of bottom-up approaches to diagnosis is for each DSM-V diagnostic workgroup to preserve the entire set of features they considered—that is, both the core clinical features they ultimately used in the categorical definition and the other clinical features they considered but chose not to use. In other words, "other clinical features" are illness manifestations considered possibly clinically relevant to a disorder but not included by the workgroup as part of the illness criteria. The workgroup process often involves debate about which candidate criteria should be part of the categorical definition. A diagnosis-specific set of "other clinical features" provides an opportunity to include the rejected candidates as possibly relevant. The final set of core criteria are meant to be exclusive; the list of "other clinical features" is meant to be inclusive. Of course there would be cross-diagnostic redundancy in this set of clinical features, just as there now is in the DSM-IV diagnostic criteria: prominent mood symptoms are included in criteria for both major depression and schizoaffective disorder, for example. But any interview based on this collection of items would eliminate redundancies: a particular symptom need only be asked once, even if used in more than one diagnosis. Collectively, these symptom items may not encompass all phenomenology potentially relevent to mental disorders, but would likely come as close as is possible, based on our current state of knowledge.

Exploration of bottom-up approaches to diagnosis would be relevant primarily to those interested in taxonomy and would not be used in making diagnoses according to DSM-V. However, ascertainment of both core and other clinical features in population surveys would permit systematic comparison of top-down and bottom-up diagnosis. The results of such comparisons would also enhance the search for diagnostic validity and would be immensely informative for future revisions of DSM.

# Conclusion

Clearly, creating dimensional scales corresponding to categorical DSM-V criteria does require guidance from the DSM Task Force, some additional effort at the workgroup level, and statistical exploration. However, the suggestions offered here have the potential to significantly improve the taxonomy for DSM's most basic and utilitarian function, the diagnosis of patients in clinical practice. Ascertaining the information necessary to give a patient a dimensional score for a particular categorical diagnosis requires virtually no additional effort of the examiner, or the patient, beyond what is already the de facto norm in clinical practice. By and large, the suggested changes simply add consistency to what most clinicians already do on their own. Taking these steps would enhance the ongoing search for diagnostic validity.

# References

Achenbach TM. Child Behavior Checklist and related instruments. In Maruish ME (ed) The Use of Psychological Testing for Treatment Planning and Outcomes Assessment, 2nd Edition. Hillsdale, NJ: Erlbaum, 1999, pp. 429–466.

Achenbach TM, Bernstein A, Dumenci L. DSM-oriented scales and statistically based syndromes for ages 18 to 59: Linking taxonomic paradigms to facilitate multitaxonomic approaches. J Pers Assess 2005; 84: 49–63.

Althoff RR, Rettew DC, Faraone SV, Boomsma DI, Hudziak JJ. Latent class analysis shows strong heritability of the child behavior checklist-juvenile bipolar phenotype. Biol Psychiatry 2006; 60(9): 903–911.

American Psychiatric Association. Diagnostic and Statistical Manual of Mental Disorders, 3rd Edition. Washington DC, American Psychiatric Association, 1980.

Bittner A, Goodwin RD, Wittchen H-U, Beesdo K, Höfler M, Lieb R. What characteristics of primary anxiety disorders predict subsequent major depressive disorder? J Clin Psychiatry 2004; 65: 618–626.

Cassano G, Rucci P, Frank E, Fagiolini A, Dell'Osso L, Shear M, Kupfer D: The mood spectrum in unipolar and bipolar disorder: Arguments for a unitary approach. Am J Psychiatry 2004; 161: 1264–1269.

Conners C. Conners' Rating Scales – Revised. New York: Multi-Health Systems, 2001.

Frank E, Cassano GB, Shear MK, Rotondo A, Dell'Osso L, Mauri M, Maser J, Grochocinski V. The spectrum model: a more coherent approach to the complexity of psychiatric symptomatology. CNS Spectr 1998; 3(4): 23–34.

Green EK, Raybould R, Macgregor S, Gordon-Smith K, Heron J, Hyde S, Grozeva D, Hamshere M, Williams N, Owen MJ, O'Donovan MC, Jones L, Jones I, Kirov G, Craddock N. Operation of the schizophrenia susceptibility gene, neuregulin 1, across traditional diagnostic boundaries to increase risk for bipolar disorder. Arch Gen Psychiatry 2005; 62: 642–648.

Haffner S. Diabetes and the metabolic syndrome—when is it best to intervene to prevent? Atheroscler Suppl 2006; 7: 3–10.

Helzer JE, Robins LN, McEvoy LT, Spitznagel EL, Stoltzman RK, Farmer A, Brockington IF. A comparison of clinical and DIS diagnoses: Physician reexamination of lay interviewed cases in the general population. Arch Gen Psychiatry 1985; 42: 657–666.

Kendell R, Jablensky A. Distinguishing between the validity and utility of psychiatric diagnoses. Am J Psychiatry 2003; 160: 4–12.

Kendler KS: Toward a scientific psychiatric nosology, strengths and limitations. Arch Gen Psychiatry 1990; 47: 969–973.

Kiernan M, Kraemer HC, Winkleby MA, King AC, Taylor CB. Do logistic regression and signal detection identify different subgroups at risk? Implications of the design of tailored interventions. Psychol Methods 2001; 6(1): 35–48.

Kraemer HC. Evaluating Medical Tests: Objective and Quantitative Guidelines. Newbury Park, CA: Sage Publications, 1992.

Maser JD, Akiskal H. Spectrum concepts in major mental disorders. Psychiatr Clin North Am 2002; 25(4): xi–xiii.

Robins E, Guze SB: Establishment of diagnostic validity in psychiatric illness: its application to schizophrenia. Am J Psychiatry 1970; 126: 983–988.

Spitzer RL, Kroenke K, Williams JB. Validation and utility of a self-report version of PRIME-MD: The PHQ primary care study. JAMA 2000; 282: 1737–1744.

Trivedi MH, Rush AJ, Wisniewski SR, Nierenberg AA, Warden D, Ritz L, Norquist G, Howland RH, Lebowitz B, McGrath PJ, Shores-Wilson K, Biggs MM, Balasubramani GK, Fava M, Team SDS. Evaluation of outcomes with citalopram for depression using measurement-based care in STAR*D: implications for clinical practice. Am J Psychiatry 2006; 163: 28–40.

Van Os J, Fahy TA, Jones P, Harvey I, Sham P, Lewis S, Bebbington P, Toone B, Williams M, Murray R. Psychopathological syndromes in the functional psychoses: associations with course and outcome. Psychol Med 1996; 26: 161–176.

van Praag HM. Two-tier diagnosing in psychiatry. Psychiatry Res 1990; 34: 1–11.

# INDEX

*Page numbers printed in **boldface** type refer to tables or figures.*